Praise for *DIY Kombucha*

This is a precious book written with a deep personal passion for
the subject; more importantly, with the conscientiousness of a caring
chef and teacher, as if present in your kitchen, walking you through
every possible nuance. This is how the world of food and health
ought to be communicated.

TONY MINICHIELLO Culinary Instructor/Co-Owner,
Northwest Culinary Academy of Vancouver

Reading *DIY Kombucha* feels as if you are sitting in one
of Andrea's classes. She brings her humor and openness to every
section, making this book an easy read that is incredibly informative
and entertaining. Even the most novice homebrewers will leave
these pages feeling confident; at the same time, experienced
brewers will find themselves taking notes.

KATE MCLAUGHLIN, R.H.N.,Owner/ManageR,
Canadian School of Natural Nutrition - Vancouver Branch

What a wonderful book! Concise, yet comprehensive and certainly
comforting to such as myself, who never had much confidence in their
kombucha brewing skills. Now, with the deeper understanding this
book provides, I feel confident to go way beyond the basics.
Thank you, Andrea, for this new empowerment!

JENNI BLACKMORE, author, *Permaculture for
the Rest of Us* and *Food Lover's Garden*

With a perfect blend of personal stories, science, and recipes, author Andrea Potter tells you everything you need to know to brew not only kombucha, but other fermented beverages as well. Even though I've been brewing kombucha for several years myself, I still learned a few things, and I can't wait to try making beet cream soda and some of the other unique fermented drinks.

DEBORAH NIEMANN ThriftyHomesteader.com, author, *Homegrown and Handmade, Ecothrifty*, and *Raising Goats Naturally*

Andrea Potter's book gives a detailed introduction to the process of making kombucha, as well as water kefir, honey-based jun, ginger beer and more. She thoroughly covers everything you need to know to get started, from equipment to sourcing ingredients, along with a primer on the science of fermentation. With plenty of photos and step-by-step instructions, *DIY Kombucha* will help you successfully make fermented beverages in your own kitchen.

VICTORIA REDHED MILLER author, *Craft Distilling, From No-Knead to Sourdough* and *Pure Poultry*.

Andrea Potter has created a wonderful resource for beginning kombucha brewers and fermented beverage enthusiasts. She delves into the history of kombucha, its health benefits, and how to master the art of kombucha making. She goes through the process step by step and offers troubleshooting.

Her book is beautifully curated with dozens of recipes including fermented beverages using medicinal herbs. It is sure to spark a love for creating your own kombucha.

CRYSTAL STEVENS author, *Grow Create Inspire* and *Worms at Work*

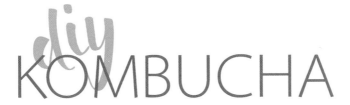

diy KOMBUCHA

sparkling homebrews made easy

ANDREA POTTER

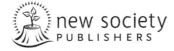

new society
PUBLISHERS

Cover design by Diane McIntosh.

@iStock main image 483925519, LID 691668260,
mason jar drink 528284756, mint sprig 682636478

Printed in Canada. First printing September 2018.

This book is intended to be educational and informative. It is not intended to
serve as a guide. The author and publisher disclaim all responsibility for any
liability, loss, or risk that may be associated with the application of any of the
contents of this book.

Any other inquiries can be directed by mail to:
New Society Publishers
P.O. Box 189, Gabriola Island, BC V0R 1X0, Canada
(250) 247-9737

LIBRARY AND ARCHIVES CANADA CATALOGUING IN PUBLICATION

Potter, Andrea, 1983-, author
    DIY kombucha : sparkling homebrews made easy / Andrea Potter.

Issued in print and electronic formats.

ISBN 978-0-86571-887-6 (softcover).—ISBN 978-1-77142-274-1 (EPUB).—
ISBN 978-1-55092-679-8 (PDF)

    1. Kombucha tea. 2. Fermented beverages. 3. Fermentation—
Amateurs' manuals. I. Title.

TP650.P68 2018   641.87'7 C2018-904198-6   C2018-904199-4

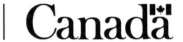

Funded by the Government of Canada   Financé par le gouvernement du Canada   Canada

New Society Publishers' mission is to publish books that contribute in funda-
mental ways to building an ecologically sustainable and just society, and to do
so with the least possible impact on the environment, in a manner that models
this vision.

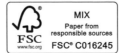

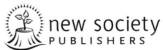

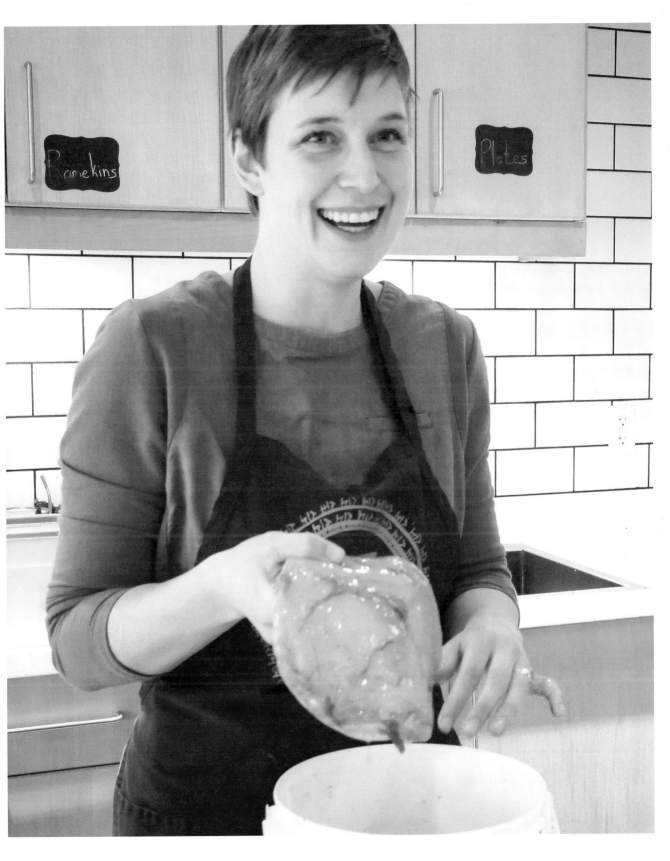

CONTENTS

THANK YOU xii

PREFACE 1

1 **AN INTRODUCTION TO HOMEBREWED SPARKLING BEVERAGES** 4

The Revival of Kombucha and Homemade Fermented Sodas 4

    Science 6

Water, Sugar, Culture 8

    Water 9

    Sugar 10

    Culture 12

Equipment 15

    Cleaning the Equipment 18

That Wobbly Line between Alcoholic and Nonalcoholic 18

Carbonation 21

    Too Much Fizz: How to
    Avoid Overcarbonation 22

    Protect Yourself and Save the Mess 24

    Too Little or No Fizz: Troubleshooting
    Lack of Bubbles 24

2 KOMBUCHA 26

What is a SCOBY? Its History
and Other Interesting Facts 26

    From Homebrewed to Store
    Shelves and Back Again 29

About the Culture 29

    Is My Brew Probiotic? 30

    Sugar 31

    Alcohol 32

Kombucha Ingredients 34

Where to Get Your First SCOBY 34

How Big a SCOBY Do You Need? 35

Tea 37

    Which Tea Will You Try? 37

Herbal Kombucha 39

Primary Fermentation: Teas and Herbs 40

What Type of Sugar to Use 42

Kombucha Basic Recipe 43

Adding Flavor and Carbonation to Your Batch 47

    Method 1: Flavor the Whole Batch 47

    Method 2: Create Different Flavors

    in Each Bottle 49

Care for Your Mother: The SCOBY Hotel 51

    Maintaining the Hotel 52

What To Do With Over-Fermented

(Vinegary) Kombucha 52

What To Do With Extra SCOBYs 54

Kombucha and SCOBY Troubleshooting 55

Kombucha as an Ingredient 57

    Mah's Orange Mint Kombucha Spritz 59

    Coconut Kefir Kombucha Smoothie 60

3   **JUN: THE HONEY-LOVING SCOBY** 62

Jun Basic Recipe 69

4   **WATER KEFIR** 72

Water Kefir Culture 72

Where to Get Water Kefir Grains 74

What to Feed Water Kefir 75

Fermenting Fruit Juices and Adding Syrups 75

Water Kefir Basic Recipe 77

Caring for Your Kefir Grains 79

Remaining Sugar and Alcohol 81

A Rhythm of Its Own 81

Coconut Kefir Yogurt Recipe 83

5 WILD-FERMENTED GINGER BEER; FRUIT AND HERBAL SODAS 86

Ginger Beer or Ginger Ale? 86

Why *Wild*-Fermented? 87

Making and Caring for a Ginger Bug 87

Ginger Beer Basic Recipe 91

Root Beer 95

    Root Beer Recipe 97

    Variations 98

        Love Your Liver Root Beer Tonic 98

        Elderberry Immunity Soda 99

        Turmeric Cardamom Fizz 101

        Beet Cream Soda 105

    Ginger Beer and Ginger Bug Fermented Soda Troubleshooting and FAQ 107

6 WHEY-FERMENTED DRINKS 110

Using Whey as a Starter for Fermented Sodas 110

How to Obtain Whey 110

Beet Kvass Recipe 112

RESOURCES 115

ABOUT THE AUTHOR 116

A NOTE ABOUT THE PUBLISHER 118

THANK YOU

I am sincerely grateful for the support that I have received from my fermentation workshop participants, comrades in fermentation geekery Cedana and Cierra, as well as friends and family for encouraging me to share this knowledge in book form. Special thanks to Kate McLaughlin and the Canadian School of Natural Nutrition, Vancouver, for permission to use the school's kitchen for the photos, to Chris and Hona for their photos, and to Catherine Pulkinghorn for guidance when I needed it most.

ANDREA

PREFACE

YOU NEVER KNOW which moments in life will create that spark—that lightning bolt of energy that illuminates a new area of fascination and then animates this interest into a quest for deeper understanding. At first it was not clear what I was chasing, but the everyday experiments bubbling away on my countertop have created (but also literally quenched) a thirst for understanding more about a vast range of topics that affect my experience of life. For me, a snapshot of such lightning moments is actually best seen in the rearview mirror. A series of seemingly mundane events led me to meeting and subsequently trying to understand my first kombucha culture, and becoming responsible for feeding this alien-looking yeast and bacteria mat, beginning a symbiotic exchange where I reap the benefits of the tasty beverage that the organism has alchemized from plain tea and sugar.

The first fermented beverage I consumed was by accident. Rummaging through a friend's pantry as a kid, I found a grape juice box. It was bulging, all the corners rounding under pressure building inside. Piercing it with the straw—*gush*—I enthusiastically guzzled the fizzy drink. My first taste of wine was very unrefined; the presence of some wild yeast had transformed the sugars in the juice box, creating carbonation and alcohol. This memory contributed to my

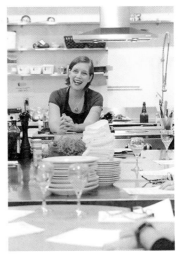

▲ Some fermented beverages at the dinner table at a cooking class the author presented. KRAUSE BERRY FARMS AND ESTATE WINERY

later understanding of wild yeast and the transformation that I was creating (this time on purpose) in making my first ginger beer.

Skipping forward a decade or so, my stepdad was on another of his health kicks. This time, he had some sort of mushroom (as he called it) growing in a big plastic bucket in the basement. He would harvest and then chug the vinegary-smelling, murky water from the bucket, referring to it as the "fountain of youth." There were rumors that kombucha could help one's hair grow back, so maybe it was *that* pillar of youth he was chasing (spoiler alert—kombucha is not a cure for male-pattern baldness). The kombucha he was brewing wasn't given the right conditions to create the tasty, slightly tangy and bubbly brew that we love, so that regime went the way of any other health fad.

The topic of fermentation came up a few years later. While tasting oils and vinegars in culinary school for garde-manger class, I stumped the teacher by asking, "But where does vinegar come from?" leading me on a tangent into food chemistry, learning about the fermentation of sugars into organic acids, and piquing my interest into the fascinating lives of micro-organisms and how they shape the flavors, nutrition, and even textures of our food.

And finally, after I had been working in restaurant kitchens for years, a coworker friend of mine (who has a talent for sourdough baking and a background in nutrition) was raving about the health benefits of this drink called kombucha, and she offered to bring some for me. I flashed back to the big plastic bucket that my stepdad brewed his powerfully vinegary health tonic in, so I politely declined to taste the stuff. Later on, while visiting her place, she handed me a glass of bubbly, slightly tangy, yeasty-smelling drink. I enthusiastically drank it, asking for more, assuming that it was some sort of homemade alcoholic cider. The feeling of radiant energy was actually not because of alcohol; it was some of that nutrition magic she had been so excited about. Now that I was finally on board and fully excited about this drink, she introduced me to the SCOBY that was responsible for making the tasty fermented tea. She showed me how to brew and sent me home with my first kombucha culture. For years now, I have been sharing the descendants of this culture, and mixing them with other cultures that I have been given, passing them on to countless friends and participants of fermentation workshops that I lead. I have also shared one with my stepdad and he's back into brewing kombucha, but this time, with much tastier results by adjusting his brewing method.

Making kombucha and other fermented beverages really satisfies the culinary nerd in me. Creating tasty and inventive flavor combinations while learning more about food science and traditional cultural food and drink is what I will spend my life being fascinated with and will pass on to my daughter, so maybe she will pick up the good fermentation bug.

Brewing drinks and fermenting jars of food has also inspired me to study holistic nutrition, with specific interest in how microbes affect and largely comprise personal health. I have made it part of my life's work to understand and befriend the bacteria that support my health, as well as learning about the role of these invisible creatures in creating and maintaining cultural diversity, resulting in strong and resilient systems (both in the micro-world and in societal cultures).

The added benefit of environmental sustainability and independence in doing it yourself (vs. depending on corporations to supply food sustenance) means that the practice of brewing my own fermented drinks is not just a fad; it is woven into daily routines that enrich my life on many levels and so is here to stay. Making my own fermented foods and drinks is a microcultural practice that is fortified every time I share the knowledge passed on to me, or whenever I pass along another SCOBY to a friend.

AN INTRODUCTION TO HOMEBREWED SPARKLING BEVERAGES

THE REVIVAL OF KOMBUCHA AND HOMEMADE FERMENTED SODAS

Welcome to the world of home-fermented beverages! Whether you have dabbled here before and need more guidance, or are just entering into your first project, this book will help you confidently craft lively, refreshing, fizzy, and healthier drinks at home.

When I embarked on my journey into fermenting beverages, I learned from a friend who was kind enough to give me my first kombucha culture (aka SCOBY) and show me how to brew. The SCOBY itself was a pancake-shaped mat floating in some murky, brownish liquid. It was tinted brown, apparently from being used to brew some black tea, and it had the texture of raw squid. It was truly unusual to me, but I was ready to take on caring for this creature so that it could in turn take care of me. On the surface, it seemed incredibly simple. Once I got my new culture home and enthusiastically brewed my first batch by making sweetened tea and cooling it to room temperature before adding the SCOBY and liquid from previous batch, I watched the kombucha culture drift around in the sweet tea in the jar. Some doubts started to intrude upon my newbie glow; I started questioning what exactly was happening in that jar. What is this SCOBY, anyway? How would I know when it was ready? Would it be obvious if it went bad? Why can I leave this on the counter for days

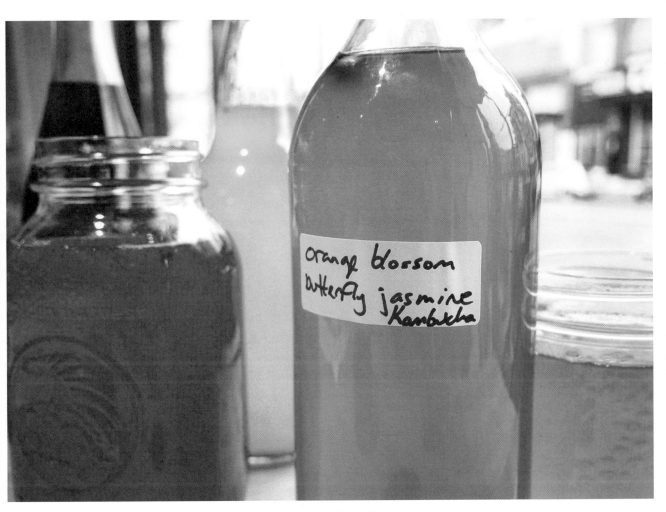

▲ A rainbow of fermented drinks: beet kvass, turmeric soda, and butterfly peaflower kombucha. HONAMI WATANABE

and weeks and it not make me sick?! So I dug deeper, looking, of course, on the internet, where I was suddenly knee-deep in zealous articles on both the "for" and "against" sides of homebrewing kombucha. After getting sucked into the research wormhole, it seemed like special equipment and know-how was necessary to brew consistent and safe beverages. It was intimidating.

Coming back to brew with my friend, who was as confident and relaxed about brewing as she was with making bread or throwing together a salad, helped me remember that we are definitely not treading new waters here. While it may be a few generations back for some of us, remembering that people have been fermenting beverages through all of civilization has helped me and my fellow fermentation enthusiasts relax and have fun as we learn. Long before we had the technology to see and subsequently name, count, and classify the micro-organisms that surround us, people have learned by observing these natural processes, and by passing on the knowledge of fermentation to each other—just as I was learning from my friend in her kitchen and have offered the skill back through workshops and now through this book.

In some traditions, fermentation is referred to as cooking without heat. Just as we have become masters of fire, knowing how applying heat to food will change the textures and flavors, so too can we harness the ancestral knowledge of how the process of fermentation works to produce new flavors, properties, and textures in our food and drink.

Science

A little science on basic beverage fermentation will help us get a handle on the seemingly mysterious world of bacteria and yeasts that transform sweet liquids into fizzy, tangy, healthier beverages. By understanding a little more about what's happening in the microcosm inside your bubbling jars and bottles, you will become a better problem solver and, therefore, a more adventurous and confident brewer. While I slept through much of my chemistry class in school, when I became fascinated with the applied science of food and beverage fermentation, suddenly my interest in science was piqued.

In culinary school, during salad dressings class, we were doing a vinegar tasting. An innocuous question sparked my quest to understand more about microbes: "But where does vinegar come from? How is it made?" My question stumped the instructor. "Well, err, it is just wine, or apple juice that is left out and goes sour…?" So my query left me sifting through chemistry formulas, starting with carbohydrates and ending up with acids.

But how? Who or what was responsible for the conversion of sugar to vinegar? The next step led me from chemistry to biology books, learning about yeast and bacterial fermentation.

I am by no measure a food scientist, but getting a handle on the basic science of fermentation in food and drinks helped me understand food safety, troubleshoot a gushing or burst bottle, a soda that didn't fizz, and get to the bottom of why one batch went differently than planned while the next was tasty.

I appreciate this straightforward definition of fermentation by Sandor Katz, author of *Wild Fermentation* and *The Art of Fermentation*: Fermentation = the transformative action of micro-organisms.

This simple definition reminds me that fermentation is all around us! It is what turns milk into yogurt, transforms flour and water into delicious sourdough bread, puts bubbles and alcohol into malted barley water to make beer, and makes sweetened tea into fizzy, sour kombucha. Fermentation is responsible for the transformation of flavors, textures, and nutrition of many of the foods and drinks we love. We are innately attracted to foods and drinks that have benefitted from the transformative process that is fermentation. As you can see, fermentation produces a wide variety of different outcomes, depending on: 1) the medium (contents of the food or drink being fermented); 2) time (how long it was cultured for); and 3) the conditions it was cultured in (like temperature, humidity, access to oxygen, etc.). People spend their lifetimes becoming craft makers of just one or a few of these foods or drinks, perfecting their methods as they learn the intricacies of the specific culture(s) at work.

While I admire that people dedicate their lives to becoming experts at a narrow scope of fermented beverages or foods, do not let this discourage you from trying your hand at it. Carrying on the craft of fermenting beverages can easily be incorporated into home kitchen routines; in fact the realm of beverage fermentation has roots in home kitchens all over the world; it was first the domain of amateur cooks, with access only to basic equipment, handed-down recipes and cultures, and hands-on learning. In this book, you'll learn about basic beverage fermentation, with a focus on low-alcohol drinks. These are projects that are right at home on any kitchen countertop or tucked away into an airy pantry.

THE BASIC FORMULA FOR FERMENTED BEVERAGES IS AS FOLLOWS

Water + sugar + micro-organisms (bacteria and/or yeasts and sometimes even mold) = Alcohol production, reduced sugar content, carbon dioxide, production of organic acids, increased enzyme activity, increased bacteria counts and production of B vitamins.

These are the key factors that contribute to how much of each product of fermentation that you get:
1. Time
2. Temperature
3. Type of organism (culture[s]) introduced
4. Amount of available sugar

Two examples:

1. A yeast-dominant culture at higher temperatures with high sugar content will result in higher alcohol and carbon dioxide production.
2. Bacteria-dominant culture over a longer period of time will result in a drink that has the least sugar, little to no alcohol, and is highly acidic (vinegary). A batch of long-fermented kombucha will accomplish this high acidity, low sugar, and alcohol.

WATER, SUGAR, CULTURE

While each beverage has its own nuances, the ingredients water + sugar + culture are constant. The quality of your inputs will make a difference for the outcome. Remember, the cultures you are caring for are living things. Give them good quality ingredients and they will thrive and perpetuate themselves. That said, fermented beverages have been made in home kitchens using what's around for centuries, so feel free to improvise and use what you have. I wouldn't canoe to a fresh spring for water to make most everyday sodas (but that does sound like a nice pace to create slow food and drink by).

I'll mention a bit about each of those ingredients here, and for each recipe, you may find that you can switch things up a bit.

Water

TIP Use the best water you have available. Purchasing a good water filter is a great investment for your health and the health of the cultures that you are growing in your fermented drinks. Look for a solid carbon block filter to install on your tap. Only ever run cold water through the block filter and change as often as is recommended.

One historical motivation for people to ferment their own drinks was to make their water safer to drink. The acids and alcohol that form during fermentation actually kill off some potentially dangerous bacteria and parasites in the water. Fermentation of drinks has resulted in safer beverages in situations with less-than-ideal water sources. Neither fermenting beverages nor boiling water removes heavy metals, though, so if the water is contaminated with lead, arsenic, or other heavy metals, switching to another water source is imperative for your health.

Whatever the water source, be sure to use clean, drinkable water. In the spirit of DIY, I refuse to buy bottled water. I am fortunate enough to live where water from the tap is clean. Even so, I choose to affix a solid block charcoal filter to my tap to minimize any potential chlorine, fluoride, lead, and other contaminants.

I know people who trek to a nearby mountain spring to get water for their drinking and brewing, claiming that the increased mineral content helps the SCOBY grow, just as the added minerals benefit their own health. The trek has become a ritual part of the making of kombucha.

TIP Traditional brewing of fermented beverages is steeped in ritual. Ritualizing everyday health-giving activities can enrich our lives by bringing intention and purpose to what we are doing. Creating even

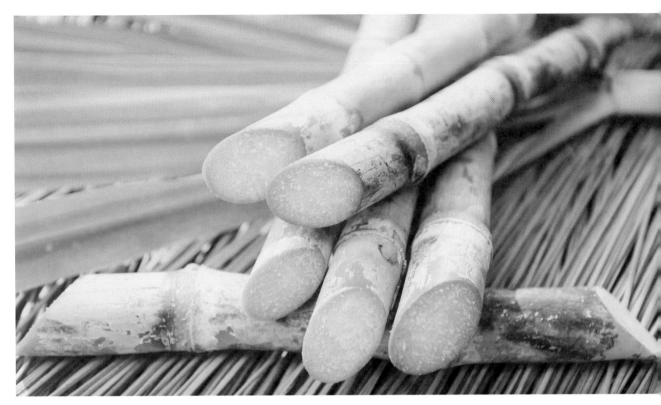

▲ Sugar cane.

a simple ritual, such as how you wash the jars and bottles, or writing positive words on the kombucha jar to imbue that batch with a desired characteristic or virtue, can bring meaning to the happiness- and health-promoting practice of making fermented drinks.

Sugar

Sugar is what drives fermentation of beverages. The yeast and bacterial cultures consume the carbohydrates, which transforms water into tasty, fizzy, sweet-sour drinks.

Best In general, the best sugar to use for fermented beverages is evaporated cane sugar. I recommend organic cane sugar to avoid both GMOs in beet sugar and residual pesticides. It can be found in well-stocked organic grocery stores. Evaporated cane juice/sugar is off-white to tan in color and is a little more granular than refined table sugar. Using organic cane sugar in fermented beverages results in a clean flavor, good, consistent carbonation, and avoidance of off-flavors that can develop from using some alternatives.

Good Refined sugar (the pure white stuff) will also produce consistent batches with a clean flavor like organic cane sugar does. In fact, I think that making refined sugar into kombucha is the only good use for the stuff. I simply avoid the extra-refined sugar because if it is labeled simply as "sugar," it is likely made from genetically modified sugar beets. I prefer to support organic agricultural practices.

Experimental I have many health-motivated students who avoid sugar in their diets, opting for alternatives such as maple syrup, fruit juices, molasses, coconut sugar, or dates—which is great for making healthier cookies, but for fermentation to work consistently well, the culture needs access to a more pure form of sugar. The presence of fiber, some minerals, and a different composition of sugars in these more wholesome sweeteners can actually interfere with fermentation, resulting in off-flavors or the culture failing to thrive. Pasteurized honey can be experimented with (⅔ cup of honey replaces 1 cup of sugar). Raw honey has its own enzymes and antibacterial properties that may compete with the culture. (With the exception of Jun, a kombucha-like drink that has adapted to love raw honey.) If you have an excess of any particular culture and want to experiment with some of the wholesome sweeteners, I encourage you to keep a fermentation journal to note what you did so you can learn what works and what doesn't.

Do not use non-caloric sweeteners! Stevia, sucralose, and sugar alcohols such as xylitol are non-caloric, and so will not feed the culture, and could actually harm it, possibly resulting in a dead SCOBY or at least a ruined batch. Agave syrup and brown rice syrup are also not recommended.

TIP The kombucha eats sugar, so you don't have to!

While I am on board with ditching the refined sugar in food and baked goods, it is important to note that kombucha and other fermented beverages require a pure source of sugar in order to ferment. The amount of sugar in the finished drink varies depending on fermenting time, temperature, and other factors, but generally the final product has between 30–80 percent less sugar than it did on the day you made it. The sugars are metabolized by the culture's resident colonies of bacteria and yeast and transformed into organic acids, B vitamins, carbon dioxide, and some alcohol.

Culture

TIP Fresh is best when you are receiving a new culture. It is okay to ask what a culture has been fed before you get one; ask about whether it was fed organic sugar and (for kombucha) tea, and whether it has been fed recently. Freeze-dried, dried, and frozen cultures will take a little more care to revive.

In this context, we're referring to the biological definition of "culture." While your motivation to craft fermented beverages might be to enjoy a refreshing drink, you are in effect actually providing the conditions for bacteria, yeast (and sometimes mold) to thrive. You are essentially a steward of these microbial cultures, and when you take care of them, they take care of you. For each project in this book, you will need the appropriate culture to get started. Under the right conditions, cultures will grow and/or multiply and so you can perpetuate your culture, sharing with friends. The kombucha, Jun, and water kefir cultures will need to be tracked down, while the ginger bug culture is a wild ferment, meaning that, like sourdough, it harnesses wild yeast and bacteria to make a fermentation starter culture.

I have been teaching fermentation classes for almost a decade now, and I estimate that I have given away well over two thousand kombucha cultures. I do brew regularly for my own consumption and a little extra for friends, which results in *lots* of kombucha SCOBYs. When I need lots of SCOBYs to send each student home with one, sometimes I call upon friends or students I have taught to brew to

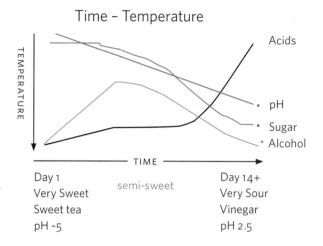

Time – Temperature

TEMPERATURE

Acids

pH

Sugar

Alcohol

TIME

Day 1	semi-sweet	Day 14+
Very Sweet		Very Sour
Sweet tea		Vinegar
pH ~5		pH 2.5

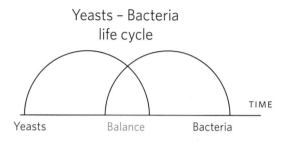

Yeasts – Bacteria life cycle

TIME

Yeasts   Balance   Bacteria

The yeast dominate until the dissolved oxygen depletes causing the yeasts to produce alcohol which fuels the bacteria to domination.

Yeast prefer cooler temperatures 60-80°F (16-27°C)
Acetro Bacteria prefer warmer 74-88°F (23-31°C)

▲ Time and temperature effect on kombucha. WWW.HAPPYHERBALIST.COM

return some of their extras so I can pass them on. Other cultures have come to me through friends who brew; my first water kefir culture came from a teacher at the nutrition school that I studied at. (I eventually neglected the water kefir grains, and attained more through Cultures for Health.)

You can order cultures online at GEM Cultures and Cultures for Health (see Resources at the end of the book). Fresh cultures may not be available for shipping outside of the US, but dried cultures can be shipped and then revived according to package instructions. Other ways of obtaining cultures are from buy/sell/swap sites, local fermentation clubs, or online groups or friends and family who brew. Passing on the physical culture becomes part of the social culture that knits us DIY folks together. Be generous by sharing your extra cultures, your tasty brewed drinks, and the knowledge of how to make them.

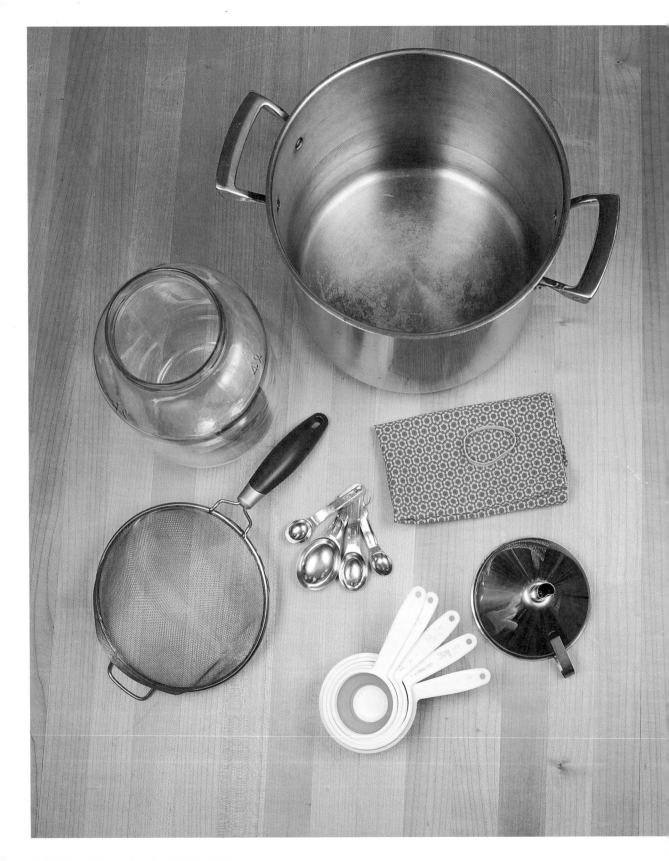

EQUIPMENT

Here are the bare bones of what you will need to make fermenting beverages fun and easy. Part of what I love about micro-batch fermenting my own drinks at home is that it is relatively easy to find what I need to get started right away. You may find what you need is already at home, or that you can get the rest from houseware or hardware stores, or rescue and reuse bottles and jars from recycling depots. Homebrew supply shops are worth a visit for some of the specialty items such as airlocks and bottling siphons. Keep an eye on buy/sell/swap websites or ads for beer or wine brewers getting rid of their equipment.

A pot (with at least 1 gallon [4L] capacity). Stainless steel or tempered glass (not aluminum).

Measuring cups and spoons.

Clear glass jars for fermenting in—1 gallon [4L] is most useful. For smaller batches, 2 quart wide-mouthed canning jars are handy. For kombucha, some people prefer a spigot for easy pouring. Just check that the nut affixing the spigot on the inside of the jar is made of hard plastic, not metal. You can sometimes get the gallon jars from delis or even hot dog carts (where they sell pickles or sauerkraut from big jars), recycle depots, or some houseware or hardware stores.

Bottles. Bail-top bottles, also known as swing-cap, are ideal. Source them from bottle depots, or buy them full of beer and drink the contents! Any colored glass should be carefully checked—some can be decorative and painted with toxic paint. Tinted glass, as in recycled beer bottles, work best. Screw-cap wine bottles can also work, as will reused store-bought kombucha bottles. You can also reuse sparkling wine/prosecco and sparkling lemonade bottles, or buy them new from a houseware or hardware store. Beware not to use square or decorative odd-shaped bottles for containing fizzy drinks, as they

> **MYTH** Using a metal spoon or strainer will harm your culture.
>
> **FACT** While prolonged contact with metal will harm the culture and potentially ruin the fermenting brew, brief contact such as stirring with a metal spoon, using tongs to lift your SCOBY, or a metal strainer to strain water kefir grains will not harm the cultures or affect your brew.

◀ Basic equipment for brewing fermented beverages.
CHRIS MCLAUGHLIN

are either more likely to explode or may not seal properly, making for a flat brew.

Funnel. You can use a plastic or metal funnel, or get a fancy one specifically for bottling, with a built-in strainer and a bevelled stem to prevent bubbling-up while pouring.

Tightly woven cloth to cover the jar, with a rubber band to secure it. Cheesecloth is not advisable, as fruit flies can get into even the smallest hole. Paper coffee filters also work fine.

Sieve/strainer. It's okay for it to have metal/wire mesh, but some people prefer nylon mesh strainers.

Wooden spoon or metal spoon/stirring implement.

The equipment below is optional but may make your production smoother, easier, or more consistent. This equipment should be available at homebrew supply shops.

A siphon. This can be simply plastic tubing or a more sophisticated siphon with a bottling attachment.

Airlocks. These are only for aging sodas and intentionally making more alcoholic drinks. Airlocks are specialized plastic or glass tubes that you fill with water, with a cork or rubber stopper for the bottle-end.

Bottle-washer attachment for tap or tiny bottle scrub brush.

Bottle-drying device such as a bottle tree.

One Step peroxide sanitizer.

▶ This equipment is optional but can make brewing more streamlined. Most equipment can be found at beer or wine brewing supply stores.
CHRIS MCLAUGHLIN

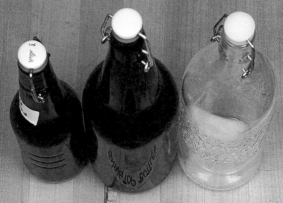

SNINGTOP BOTTLES

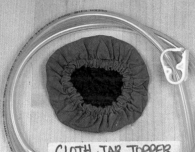

CLOTH JAR TOPPER

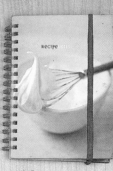

JOURNAL

AIRLOCK

HYDROMETER

BOTTLE SCRUB BRUSH

BOTTLE FILLER

FINE NYLON STRAINER

SIPHON

Hydrometer. A tool that measures how much alcohol/sugar remains in your batch.

Cleaning the Equipment

TIP It is important to remember that the fermentation processes at work on your beverages are pro-bacterial. You want to clean the equipment that comes in contact with your beverages to assure that the right types of microbes are invited to your fermentation party. Unlike in the homebrewing of beer and wine, it is not necessary to sterilize the equipment with surgical precision.

General "clean-dishes" rules apply, so hot, soapy water and a good rinse is fine for all jars, bottles, strainers, siphons, etc. Some people prefer to use a sterilizer, to avoid tedious rinsing of soapy suds. You can sterilize by using boiling water, but only on shatter-resistant glass bottles and jars; I recommend a peroxide sanitizer. You can get this in powder form and add water to it each time you brew or bottle. The peroxide sanitizer I use is called One-Step and leaves no residue or chemicals, so you don't even have to rinse it, and it is safe for your skin.

Bottles can be a pain to clean. You can get bottle-washing attachments for your tap, or use a tiny bottle scrub brush to remove any stuck-on residue before your final rinse. Depending on how big your homebrewing operation is, you may want to get a bottle drying tree as well.

THAT WOBBLY LINE BETWEEN ALCOHOLIC AND NONALCOHOLIC

TIP The life of yeast: yeast eats sugar, burps carbon dioxide, and pees out alcohol.

Albeit a little oversimplified, this goofy adage was given to me by a student at a fermentation workshop, and it is a handy reminder about the role of yeast in fermentation. Too much alcohol? Those yeasts were either fed too much sugar, or were in too high of a concentration relative to bacteria, or were a little too warm. Not enough fizz? Feed those yeasts some more sugar and make sure the "burps" are trapped.

Once I had a grasp on fermenting kombucha, I tried my hand at making ginger beer and root beer. I applied the same principle of leaving the tea with the culture in an open container to ferment for a while before bottling it. My understanding was that, as for kombucha, the longer the sweet medium fermented in the open container, the less sugar it would have, and the more benefits I would reap from the resulting brew.

And wow—did those batches pack a punch! I had accidentally created pretty strongly alcoholic root beer. I had to go back to the drawing board about what I thought I knew about fermenting drinks and here's what I learned.

In North America, government regulatory bodies have drawn a definite line between "alcoholic" and "nonalcoholic." Any fermented beverage that is sold as nonalcoholic, or is assumed not to be alcoholic will not exceed 0.5 percent alcohol. In your kitchen, the production of alcohol will not be as carefully regulated, and a brew may become a little (or a lot) more alcoholic.

Yeasts are responsible for carbon dioxide (that fizz factor we all love) as well as alcohol (ethanol) production.

Kombucha, water kefir, and wild fermented beverages use different cultures to ferment the sugars we supply them with. These cultures are comprised of communities of micro-organisms which include both bacteria and yeasts. In the production of modern beer and wine, the fermentable sugars are only acted upon by very specific alcohol-producing yeasts. Other organisms are eliminated by means of pasteurization or chemical sterilization before yeast is introduced. In contrast to beer and wine, the fermented beverages we are creating here are lower in alcohol because of the bacterial fermentation that follows the yeast fermentation.

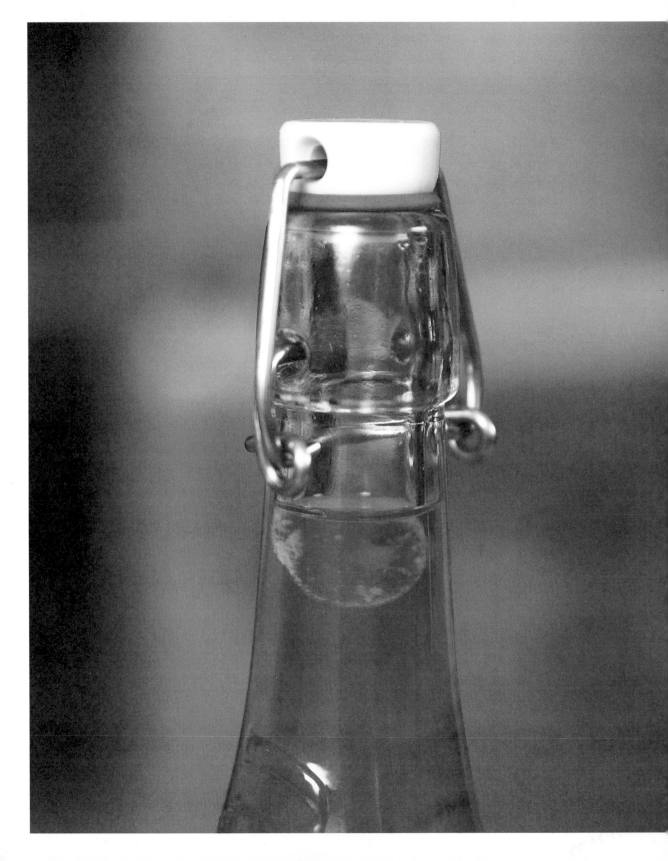

All fermented beverages produce alcohol at some stage in their fermentation. The more yeast activity, the more alcohol potential there is (and certain strains of yeast can produce very high amounts of alcohol; the more sugar you feed them the more alcohol they make). Drinks with very little alcohol and more health benefits do indeed produce alcohol during fermentation, but the next phase of fermentation reduces their alcohol content, as bacteria that are also present in the culture feed on the alcohol and produce acids.

To get back to my unintentionally alcoholic root beer project: the culture I used to create the root beer was a ginger bug. It had a lot of yeast activity, and fermenting it in an open container for a number of days, paired with warm summertime temperatures and high sugar content, created perfect conditions to make alcohol. I have modified my brewing method by reducing the sugar content somewhat and bottling the root beer or ginger beer right away after adding the culture, fermenting it only in the bottle and not in the open jar. The result is an ultra-fizzy (beware) but lower alcohol (kid-friendly) summertime sipper.

CARBONATION

TIP The results of fermentation are indeed more nuanced and varied than the shortcut method of carbonating water and adding sugar syrup. The flavors and health benefits that you are able to produce using microbial cultures and traditional methods make it all worth the effort.

Many homebrewers have a fantastic and sometimes scary tale of popped caps, geysering pressure releases, and even exploding bottles.

I'll share one such story. After I had learned how to make kombucha, I invited a friend to embark on making ginger beer with me. Our kombucha had reliable fizz, and actually aged well in the bottles (we were not doing secondary fermentation so the sugar level was low),

◀ SCOBY formation in the bottle.
CHRIS MCLAUGHLIN

making it practical to make a large batch and store the bottles for a while before enjoying them. Once we learned how to make a ginger bug, we got ambitious and thought that we'd make a summer's worth of ginger beer at once.

A couple of weeks later, my friend called me in a panic—the bottles, stacked a few cases high, had begun to explode! The only advice I could offer was to get out of the line of fire, and as she took shelter, she heard one explosion detonate the others. Needless to say, it was a mess of epic proportions. Luckily, nobody got hurt.

Another story was shared over a fermentation forum that I contribute to. This unfortunate situation was costly: A bottle of half-consumed kombucha was left in a hot car while the owner was on holiday. There, in the long-term parking lot at the airport, the interior of the car got very hot, which resulted in a pressure release from the bottle—blowing the swing-cap off the bottle with such force that it shattered the car windshield!

Remember that carbonation is the work of yeast digesting sugar, which yields carbon dioxide, so beware of overcarbonated bottles!

Now that I have illustrated that overcarbonation can cause serious damage, let's learn from these mistakes.

Too Much Fizz: How to Avoid Overcarbonation

Fill bottles to halfway up the neck (almost full). Underfilled bottles can pressurize incredibly, as carbon dioxide fills the space in the bottle.

Do not shake bottles! Those yeast love oxygen, so don't overexcite them. Warm temperatures increase yeast activity, so don't put sealed bottles in the warmest area of the house. Comfortable room temperatures (66–77°F [19–25°C] for most beverages) are ideal for fermenting beverages, and fridge or cold-storage (39–50°F [4–10°C]) slow down fermentation, so store carbonated bottles in cold-storage.

Burp your bottles. Carefully open them during fermentation and listen to the pressure release. Once you get sufficient pressure, move

▶ Carefully opening a very fizzy bottle. CHRIS MCLAUGHLIN

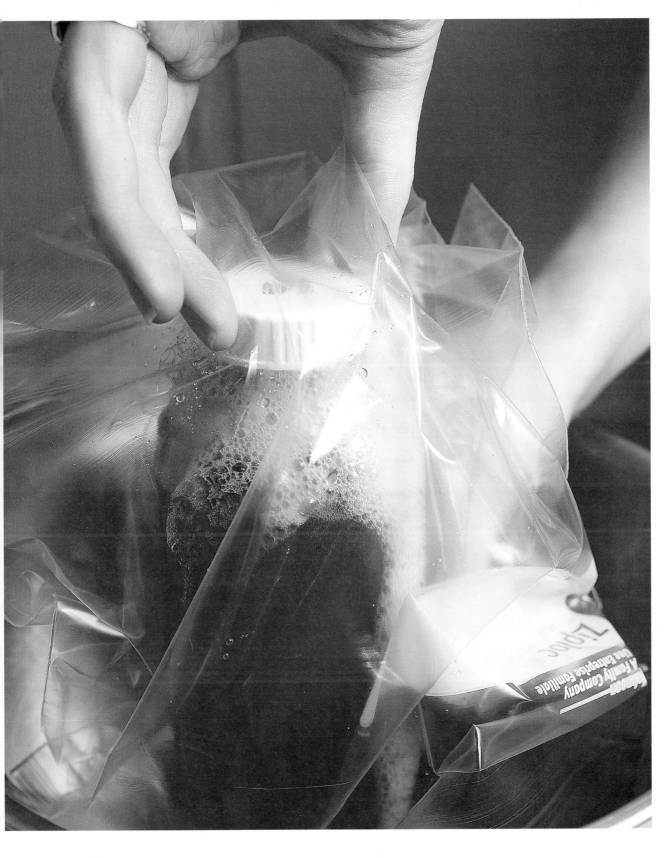

the bottles into the fridge. The fridge slows fermentation, but does not completely stop it, so I recommend drinking your beverages within a month or so.

Protect Yourself and Save the Mess

I have resorted to using a big plastic bin with a lid to store fermenting beverages. (I refer to this setup as "the bomb shelter.")

Open bottles carefully. One trick that I found is to put the bottle in a big bowl, put a plastic bag over the cap and neck of the bottle as you slowly open the swing-top bottle. Any geyser is prevented from staining your ceiling and the excess is just poured into your glass once the fizz dies down.

Too Little or No Fizz:
Troubleshooting Lack of Bubbles

Once you have bottled your beverage and are finding that you get little to no carbonation, check these things and adjust:

Do your bottles seal properly? The best bottles to use are swing-cap bottles that are designed to hold in carbonation. Used beer bottles or prosecco bottles or bottles bought specifically for fermenting drinks are ideal for holding in fizz. Check the gasket for integrity of the seal and replace if needed.

Culture not active? If you used a kombucha or water kefir SCOBY or ginger bug, you may need to replace it.

Not enough sugar or the wrong type of sugar? Yeast needs easy-to-digest sugar, so experimental sugars might result in slow fermentation and few bubbles.

Too cold? Move to a warmer spot. I place the bottled bevvies in my oven with the light on for a couple of days if I want more bubbles and am getting impatient.

Very few bubbles? You can gently swirl the bottles around a bit, move them to a warmer spot and keep waiting for the carbonation to happen. Never forget about your bottles though, as they can go from too little to too much carbonation within a few days.

2

KOMBUCHA

WHAT IS A SCOBY? ITS HISTORY AND OTHER INTERESTING FACTS

▶ SCOBY suspended in black tea kombucha. CHRIS MCLAUGHLIN

KOMBUCHA IS A sparkling fermented beverage, made with tea and sugar, that has very deep roots. It has been documented as far back as 200 BC, during the Qin Dynasty in China, where it was brewed as a longevity elixir.

Kombucha is known the world over by many different names. Translated as variations of "tea mushroom/bacteria/fungus/yeast," "tea of immortality," "hero mushroom," "sea treasure," "stomach treasure." just to name a few, the name "kombucha" has its own story. It is said that a Korean doctor by the name of Dr. Kombu brought this tea to Japan, impressing Emperor Inyko in 414 AD. *Cha* is Chinese for tea and many cultures use a similar word for that drink.

It is also said that Samurai warriors carried the elixir in their wineskins, giving them energy and courage for battle.

The brew made its way to Europe through Russia before making a big splash in North America by the 1960s, with surges in popularity all over the world ever since. Jars of sweet tea with a mysterious jellyfish-like culture floating around in it have graced countertops and home fermentation shacks the world over. Kombucha has proud homebrewing roots.

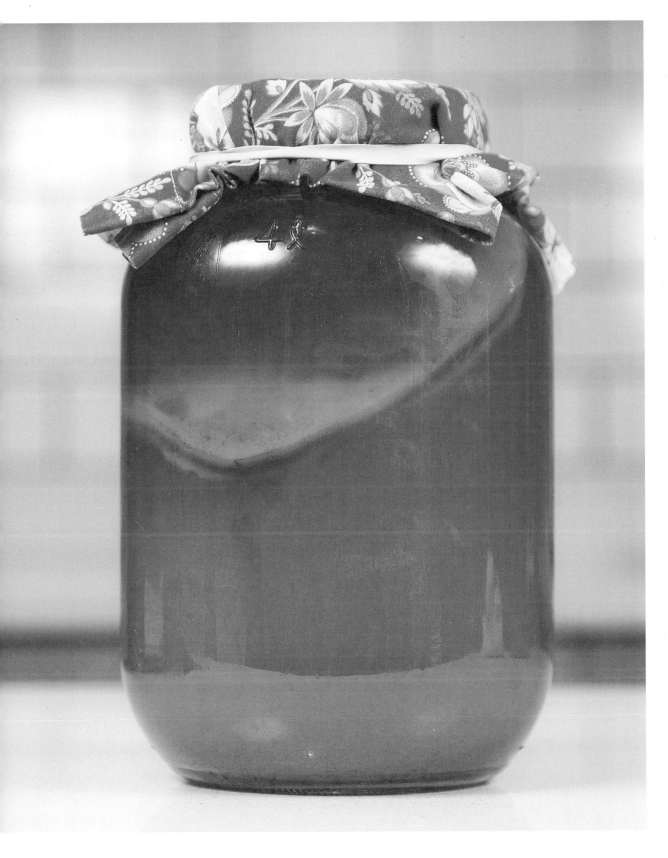

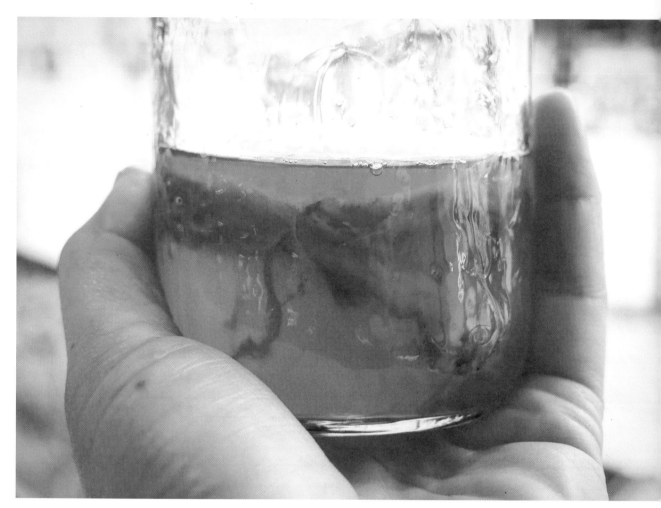

▲ Kombucha SCOBY. HONAMI WATANABE

During a kombucha workshop I am teaching, someone inevitably asks, "But where did the first one come from?" Incredibly, the actual physical origin of the kombucha SCOBY is as shrouded in myth and mystery as the name is. One origin story with good potential to have some truth in it is that it is derived from a parasitic fungus that grows on birch trees, feeding off the sap. (Another name for kombucha includes "birch mushroom.") How and why an ancient human came across that tree fungus, observed its thirst for sugar, and took it home as a "pet" who would brew a tasty beverage in exchange for nutrients, is mysterious indeed. Herbal and natural medicine traditions have arisen from traditional peoples' deep connection as part of nature, and so perhaps the culture "spoke" to certain humans and told them how to brew the healing tea.

From Homebrewed to Store Shelves and Back Again

The effervescent, tangy tea drink has hit another peak in popularity in North America, largely due to the fact that the beverage industry has finally caught on to the trend, classifying kombucha as a leader in the exploding "functional beverage" sector. Big business has had many trials and tribulations in taming the SCOBY enough to make consistent batches. Unlike beverages made with isolated microbes, such as most beer and wine, the factors of alcohol production, carbonation, and acidity in kombucha can vary from batch to batch and from culture to culture. Although kombucha brewers on large and small commercial scales have managed to get the good stuff into bottles, and have been experimenting with some really great flavors, I still think that the wildness of kombucha should be celebrated, not tamed. It lends itself best to homebrewed microbatches and plenty of experimentation with flavors from different teas, herbs, fruits, and other fun flavoring ingredients.

ABOUT THE CULTURE

Kombucha is brewed by a unique culture, usually referred to as a SCOBY (which is an acronym for Symbiotic Culture of Bacteria and Yeast), also lovingly called the Mother (similar to mother of vinegar, a pellicle that forms in fermenting vinegar, but different because the kombucha SCOBY is home to yeast and not only bacteria). How kombucha has traveled the world is by the interesting way it reproduces. Unlike most other yeast and bacterial cultures, kombucha forms a thin layer—the SCOBY—which is a cellulose mat. With each batch of sweet tea that it ferments, it grows and reproduces. If you hear of any

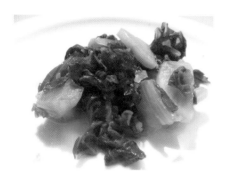

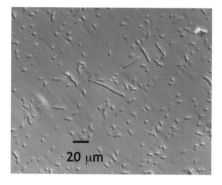

▲ Kimchi

~1.9 x 107 CFU/ml *

Lactobacillus
Leuconostoc
Weissella

* Chang, Ji Yoon, and Hae Choon Chang (2011) Journal of food science 76.1: M72-M78.

ESPERANZA GARCIA

talk in the kombucha brewer's community about Mother and Daughter or Baby cultures, they are referring to the original SCOBY that fermented the tea and the new SCOBY that resulted from the fermentation. I don't use the terms Mother and Daughter/Baby, because it can be confusing, and since there is no Father culture, it's also inaccurate. As the microbes consume the sugar, they replicate, so the SCOBY is actually cloning itself.

The yeasts and bacteria in the SCOBY act on the nitrogen, tannins, and phenolic compounds in the tea and the carbohydrates in sugar to produce acetic, gluconic, and butyric acids, and sometimes lactic acid (from probiotic bacteria *Lactobacilli*). These acids are powerful aids in the body's cleansing process. In addition to these organic acids, kombucha creates B vitamins during fermentation. It is consumed as a natural energy booster, digestive aid, and liver-cleansing beverage.

Is My Brew Probiotic?

Probiotic is defined by the World Health Organization (2001) as "live micro-organisms which, when administered in adequate amounts, confer a health benefit on the host."

There is debate about whether the kombucha fermentation produces probiotic bacteria. Now that larger studies have been done on kombucha, thanks to its explosion in popularity, analysis is showing varied results. While *Lactobacilli* are classified as probiotic bacteria, and some kombucha cultures do contain these bacteria, others do not. Keep in mind that only certain studied strains of micro-organisms are currently classified as probiotic. Micro-organisms are continually being discovered that are found to benefit our health. It is estimated that we have only actually discovered and classified about ten percent of the earth's microbiome. As I write this, scientists from all over the world are finding and classifying more micro-organisms, with the lofty goal of discovering all of the microbes that live on earth. With all of this still to be discovered, I am anticipating a day when we know more about the biodiverse microbes that are present in the cultures we use to ferment delicious beverages, and I expect that we will find that more and more of these microbes actually do confer a benefit to human health.

TIP How much is too much of a good thing? While scientific analysis is catching up with identifying the fascinating and complex composition of the SCOBY and kombucha, along with which components of the drink could be responsible for reported health benefits, kombucha drinkers are united in following their taste buds and listening to their guts. When it comes to knowing the right amount for you to drink, I encourage you to do the same, starting small (four ounces or so with food) and gradually adding more kombucha if you have a thirst for it. Because kombucha has liver-cleansing properties and affects the balance of organisms in your gut, too much kombucha could look like bloating, gas (which is temporary), and possibly liver-cleansing symptoms such as skin flare-ups or fatigue.

My stance on consumption of kombucha is that no, we should not rely only on kombucha to supply the beneficial microbes we need to maintain good health, just as we should not rely solely on any one cultured food or beverage. Kombucha is one of many fermented foods and beverages that can be enjoyed in moderation, contributing to the diversity of micro-organisms in our diet.

Sugar

How much sugar is in kombucha? The initial sugar in an eight-ounce glass of the sweetened tea, unfermented is 1.65 ounces. After seven days of fermentation at average room temperature, this reduces to 0.6 ounces (a little less than orange juice). After twenty-one days of fermentation, this reduces to 0.3 ounces (about the same as carrot juice). Factors such as the type of sugar used and the temperature in fermentation vary the resulting sugar content.

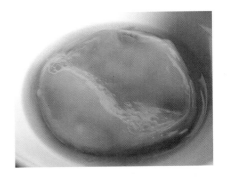

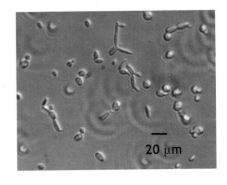

▲ Kombucha

~ 2.6 x 10⁶ CFU/ml **
Acetobacter
Gluconacetobacter
Lactobacillus
Lactococcus
Gluconobacter

~ 2.8 x 10⁶ CFU/ml
Schizosaccharomyces
Saccharomycodes
Saccharomyces
Zygosaccharomyces

** Markov et al (2012)
Archives of Biological Sciences, 64(4),
1439-1447

ESPERANZA GARCIA

Alcohol

How much alcohol kombucha produces is a hotly discussed topic. Since kombucha has become by far the most popular commercially produced fermented beverage, the amount of alcohol in kombucha sold in stores is tightly monitored and regulated. As we know from basic fermentation principles, the factors of yeast and sugar, as well as fermentation time and temperature determine the alcohol content. In kombucha, we also consider bacterial fermentation, since the bacteria consume some of the alcohol the yeast makes, resulting in a more acidic and less alcoholic drink. So the point at which you consume the kombucha also matters.

The most alcohol is produced a few days into fermentation, then the alcohol content decreases as acidity increases, so some people use a pH test to know when their kombucha has the least alcohol. I have found that relying on my taste buds works just as well; our tongues are well outfitted to detect sourness, so once your kombucha is souring, it will be lower in alcohol than the initial still-sweet and a-little-fizzy phase.

Homebrewed kombucha produces 0.5–2.5 percent alcohol. Store-bought kombucha that is sold without an alcohol warning is limited to 0.5 percent which is so little that it is considered to be nonalcoholic.

When companies started to capitalize on the kombucha trend, some got themselves in hot water with class-action lawsuits regarding the alcohol content. Secondary fermentation also increases alcohol production, and some companies were accidentally exceeding the legal amount of permitted alcohol once the bottles reached the customers. The result has been that some commercially bottled kombuchas actually have to label the bottle as alcoholic, and others are using very specific lab-selected strains of SCOBYs to have better control over the process. Still others have opted to pasteurize their kombucha, effectively stopping additional fermentation and also killing off any potentially beneficial bacteria.

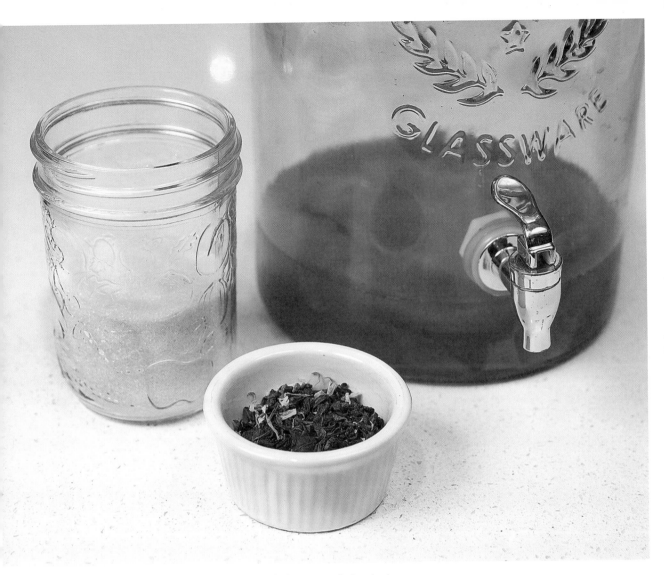

▲ Organic cane sugar and some nice jasmine and herb green tea for kombucha.
CHRIS MCLAUGHLIN

My opinion is that kombucha lends itself best to home or micro-brewed batches. To honor its wild composition and the symbiosis that exists between the organisms in the SCOBY, I keep mixing my batches up from time to time with SCOBYs I get from friends, so they can mingle organisms and stay strong in their micro-biodiversity.

KOMBUCHA INGREDIENTS

TIP Good inputs = good results, so it is best to use tea or herbs that are free from pesticide sprays.

As with most drinks with homemade origins, there are a myriad of kombucha recipes, with each homebrewer tweaking and customizing their own. There is diverse opinion within the kombucha-brewing community about what the best ingredients are to make a tasty batch, as well as to maintain good health for the SCOBY that is hard at work transforming the sweetened tea. The biggest disagreement seems to be whether green tea or black tea is best. I have used both, switching between them with successful batches that resulted in tasty kombucha as well as healthy SCOBYs.

I like observing how different people have different brewing styles. Just as you'd walk around a community garden and see many different ways of tending a plot, you will notice that folks have more or less regimented structure in their brewing practices. My friend Laurin did a more controlled experiment compared to my style of brewing different teas with the same SCOBY. I gave her two SCOBYs, and she carefully brewed two jars of kombucha, side-by-side, for a couple of years. One was with green tea and the other with black tea, keeping each SCOBY separate. I was invited over to help her harvest her SCOBYs so that I could give them to some workshop participants. Both SCOBYs were solid-looking, thick, reproducing well, and showing all the signs of a healthy culture. Both batches resulted in consistently tasty kombucha. The only visible difference was that the SCOBY that brewed the black tea was stained brown while the green tea SCOBY was more whitish.

WHERE TO GET
YOUR FIRST SCOBY

The popularity of kombucha has spanned much of the earth, with each SCOBY reproducing after a batch or two of fermentation and then being passed from one homebrewer to the next, often along with the tradition of how to brew, according to the source of the SCOBY.

Sourcing the kombucha culture may be as easy as ringing up a friend who will enthusiastically share their culture with you. If you live somewhere that does not have a visible and vibrant kombucha-brewing community, you may need to dig deeper. Turning to the internet, of course, is one way to connect with an active community of homebrewers. People give (and sometimes sell for a small to moderate fee) their excess SCOBYs on websites and buy/sell/trade platforms. Some people send them by mail, or you can often find people brewing in your area. A fresh SCOBY in at least one cup of kombucha liquid is what you're looking for.

There are also labs that culture them specifically for sale. (See Resources.) Some SCOBYs are sold dried; these take an extra step of rehydrating (according to the lab's instructions) before they are ready to ferment your first batch. I have had quite a few emails and queries about successfully bringing back dried SCOBYs. They do not seem to brew as reliably as the fresh cultures.

Kombucha can be brewed from smaller SCOBYs, and can even be cultivated from a bottle of store-bought or homemade kombucha drink. To cultivate a SCOBY from a bottle of kombucha, simply pour a bottle of plain kombucha into a clean jar, place a tightly woven cloth or paper towel over top and fix it in place with a rubber band or Mason jar ring. Let it sit at room temperature until it forms a SCOBY (this sometimes takes a few weeks). Use this SCOBY and the sour kombucha to start a new batch.

HOW BIG A SCOBY
DO YOU NEED?

The answer to this is: it depends. For a one gallon (4 L) batch, a small-ish or thin SCOBY along with the one cup of strong starter tea will be sufficient. The important thing to remember is that yeasts can double every hour with enough food (sugar) and in comfortable

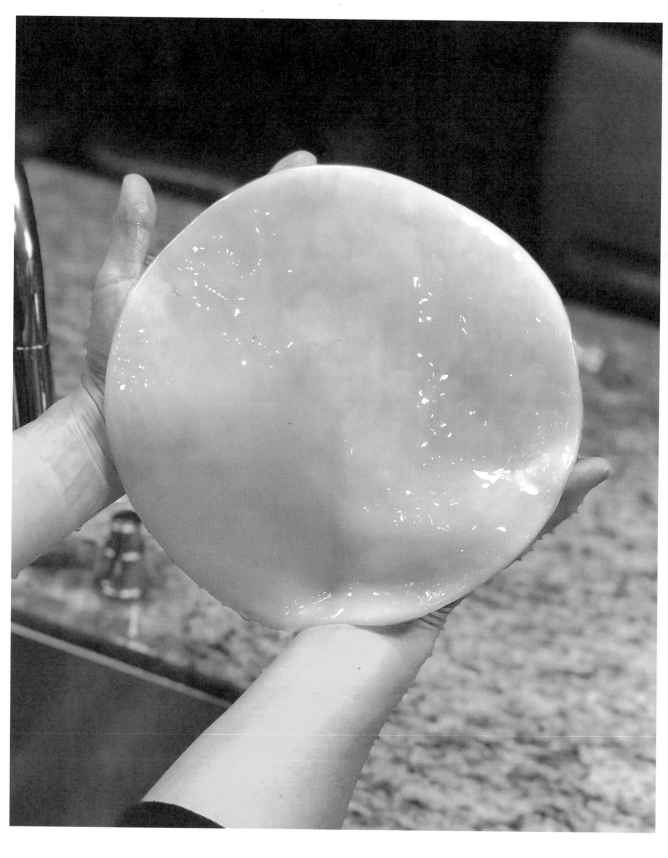

temperatures. So whether you use a huge or a relatively small SCOBY is just a matter of the batch taking a little less or a little more time to brew.

TEA

Kombucha is traditionally made with tea (*Camellia sinensis*). The type of tea it is made with affects the flavor and character of the kombucha. I recommend using only organic tea (and herbs), or tea that is not sprayed with pesticides. Both tea bags and loose leaf teas work. The earlier understanding of kombucha was that caffeine was necessary to keep the SCOBY healthy. Some information being passed around even suggested that the caffeine was metabolized by the kombucha culture, resulting in little to no caffeine. This has since been disproved. The kombucha does not metabolize the caffeine, so there is exactly as much in the finished kombucha as there was in the initial batch of sweetened tea. And, interestingly, it turns out that the kombucha SCOBY does not require caffeine at all.

In addition to sugar, the necessary ingredients for the SCOBY to thrive are contained in tea leaves: tannins, phenolic compounds, and nitrogen. Homebrewers have successfully used decaffeinated tea as well as experimenting with herbs other than tea.

Which Tea Will You Try?

Black tea contains more purines, and if you make a strong black tea kombucha, it will encourage more yeast activity, making a fizzier brew. Black tea also contains more fluoride, which is toxic in high doses, than green tea does. Sourcing quality tea is the best way to find black teas with least fluoride.

Some people like green tea for its clean, almost apple cider-like taste.

Oolong tea lovers will find the toasty notes come through in the final tea very nicely.

Earl Grey seems contentious among brewers. Some say the oil of bergamot, which is responsible for its citrusy-floral aroma and taste,

◀ They call this one "King SCOBY"! Some SCOBYS form uniform and white, some look a little less "perfect," but are still healthy. ELLA MAH

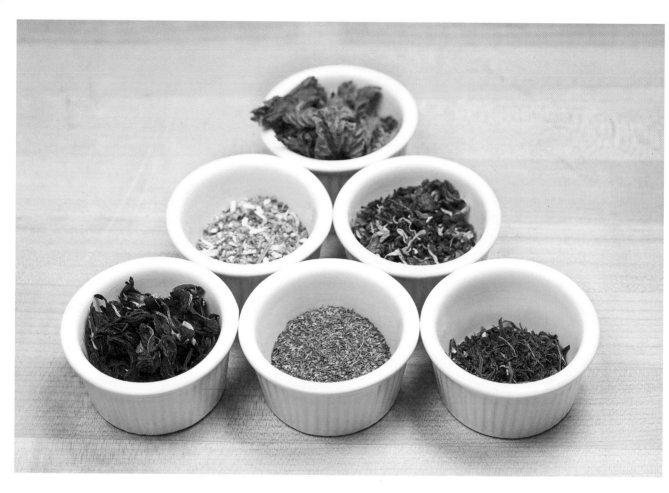

▲ Herbs for primary kombucha fermentation. CHRIS MCLAUGHLIN

is too harsh on the SCOBY. I have found that rotating through the odd batch of organic Earl Grey tea has not affected my SCOBY, and I enjoy the taste immensely. A tea merchant who I talked to mentioned that their quality Earl Grey is made with bergamot flowers, not the oil (a cheaper way to get more floral aroma), and so is far less antibacterial than cheaper Earl Grey teas, so he brews kombucha successfully with this Earl Grey.

I save the more expensive white teas for fancier brews, made for special occasions. My favorite so far has been white tea kombucha with a few sprigs of lavender added.

Flavored teas can work well too. On one visit to the tea shop, I reveled in the heady aromas of a dozen or more jars of tea before I settled on a coconut green tea. Toasted pieces of coconut were nestled in with the long strands of dried tea leaves, and the smell was of coconut macaroons! The kombucha made with it was phenomenal. It was clean and refreshing, and needed absolutely nothing more than to be enjoyed over ice in the garden. My friend often brews with a mango black tea (you can make this by adding dried mango pieces to the steeping tea) and my stepdad faithfully uses blackcurrant flavored black tea in his brew. When I use flavored teas, I usually skip the secondary fermentation step. I find that no added flavor is needed, and I enjoy some batches less fizzy. If you want a very fizzy batch of flavored tea kombucha, you can just age it in the bottle (without adding any extra sugar).

HERBAL KOMBUCHA

Now that we know that the kombucha SCOBY is not just a tea lover, we can try using different herbs instead. Whether you are avoiding caffeine altogether, or trying to include more herbs for their nutritional and therapeutic properties, kombucha is a wonderful way to integrate more herbs into your life.

I recommend talking to an herbalist to be sure that you are using herbs that are safe and beneficial for you. The science of the effects of kombucha fermentation on herbs is still new. Preliminary studies show that there is a wildly varied effect on the herbs after fermentation compared to when they are simply brewed as infusions. Some herbs increased in antioxidant levels after kombucha fermentation, while other herbs showed lower antioxidant levels. There is much to learn in this area, so for now I recommend sticking to moderate amounts of generally safe herbs for your kombucha, using tea as the tried and true brewing method for kombucha. Since tea is what has been traditionally used in kombucha, most of my batches are with tea. I sometimes add herbs or do the odd herb-only infusions.

If you require or prefer non-tea, totally noncaffeinated drinks, water kefir may be a better fit for you.

I recommend a few herbs that I have tried with success below.

PRIMARY FERMENTATION:
TEAS AND HERBS

NOTE Herbs are medicine. It is wise to consult someone knowledgeable about herbs before adding a significant amount of a specific herb to your diet. The herbs here are largely nutritive herbs, (and some are just super fragrant or a pretty color) and are generally safe in moderation. Herbs can be grown and harvested or foraged yourself or you can get them at natural food and herb shops as well as herbal apothecaries.

HERB	MEASUREMENT FOR 1-GALLON (4L) BATCH	NOTES
Hibiscus flowers	¼ cup	Noted for its vibrant red color and high vitamin C content, hibiscus flowers brew a tangy-tart kombucha.
Nettle (stinging nettle), dried	⅓–½ cup, packed	A great way to get this bitter-tasting but super-nutritive herb into your diet. I combine mine with mint for a nice flavor.
Red raspberry leaf, dried	⅓–½ cup, packed	This bland-tasting tea is a fine base for kombucha. I recommend adding a secondary fermentation flavor or another aromatic herb for flavor. This famed nutritive tea acts as a uterine strengthener.
Rooibos	1–2 heaping tablespoons (or 4–8 tea bags)	"Red tea" is high in antioxidants and makes a robust and tasty kombucha with beautiful auburn tones.
Yerba Mate	1–2 heaping tablespoons (or 4–8 tea bags)	Not everyone's cup of tea. But if you love the smokiness of yerba mate, you'll love it in kombucha.

Butterfly pea flowers, dried	⅓ cup	This craze has swept the tea world lately. Butterfly pea flowers are grown in Thailand and a few of these make the tea as blue as the sky on a clear day. The kombucha fermentation process turns it to purple for a unique and beautiful tea. I add lavender to mine for astoundingly good kombucha.
Lavender flowers, dried	¼ cup	Heady, floral aromatherapy in a bubbling glass. Use alone or combine with a tea or a complimentary herb.
Mint, dried	½ cup	Zing! This refreshing kombucha will wake you up. There are many kinds of mint, so go ahead and experi-mint.
Mint, fresh	1½ cups, loosely packed leaves	
Lemon balm, dried	½ cup	This cousin of mint grows like a weed and smells intensely lemony. It tastes a bit bitter, but I find kombucha to be a good application for it.
Lemon balm, fresh	1½ cups, loosely packed leaves	

COFFEE KOMBUCHA

Yes coffee kombucha, known as *koffucha*, has a small but fervent fan base.

I love a nice hot cuppa in the morning. I also like a tall, chilled glass of kombucha. However, I personally do not like koffucha. I would compare the taste to cold coffee with some apple cider vinegar dumped into it. But, to each their own.

Making koffucha is similar to making kombucha, but because coffee is already acidic, you do not need a starter (kombucha from a previous batch). Use a spare SCOBY for the coffee kombucha. It will stain and taste like coffee from here on.

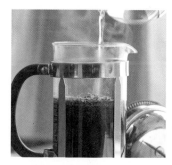

▲ Coffee beans infusing in a French press.

1. Pour 2 quarts hot coffee into a clean jar; add ½ cup sugar, stirring to dissolve.
2. Cool to room temperature and add SCOBY. Ferment as with kombucha (covered with a cloth cover, undisturbed at room temperature for a week) and start checking the taste. Once it's tasty to you, pour off the liquid and drink or refrigerate.

WHAT TYPE OF SUGAR TO USE

The fermentation process by the yeasts and bacteria consumes the sugar (so you don't have to), so feeding it a pure form of sugar actually makes for a healthier culture, resulting in healthier and tastier kombucha. Refined cane sugar works well. I choose fair-trade and organic refined sugar.

Some folks feed their kombucha a more whole form of cane sugar, such as sucanat or rapadura sugar. While some people swear by the less-refined sugar as there are minerals present in them, I have found that the resulting kombucha does not brew as quickly or as consistently as it does by using refined sugar. I encourage you to experiment with them, but I have chosen to save these more unrefined sugars for healthier baking.

Other sugars such as maple syrup and coconut sugar are also not recommended. The SCOBY needs a pure form of sucrose. Other sugars (higher in fructose) are harder for the SCOBY to metabolize, resulting in slow-to-start kombucha brews. Too slow a start to fermentation can leave the SCOBY vulnerable to other bacteria and molds, which may ruin the brew and the SCOBY.

There is a relative of kombucha called Jun which is adapted to feeding off of honey. So if you prefer to use honey, see Chapter 3 for more on Jun.

The basic recipe calls for caffeinated tea. If you want to try alternatives to tea, see the chart on pages 40–41 for suggestions of other herbs and the amounts to add instead of tea, or in addition to the tea.

1. Brew a pot of sweetened tea:
   Boil water, add sugar and tea.

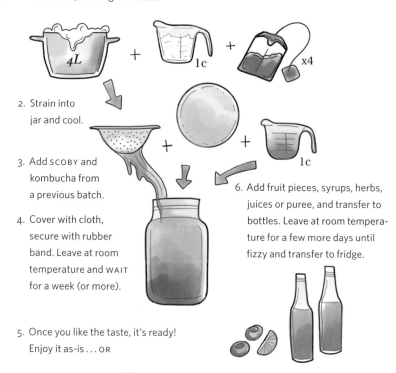

2. Strain into jar and cool.

3. Add SCOBY and kombucha from a previous batch.

4. Cover with cloth, secure with rubber band. Leave at room temperature and WAIT for a week (or more).

5. Once you like the taste, it's ready! Enjoy it as-is . . . OR

6. Add fruit pieces, syrups, herbs, juices or puree, and transfer to bottles. Leave at room temperature for a few more days until fizzy and transfer to fridge.

▲ How to make kombucha. CRYSTAL ALEXANDRIA

Makes 1 gallon (4L)
Time: 10–15 minutes prep
   (plus cooling time)
Fermentation: 7–14+ days

EQUIPMENT
Pot (1 gallon or bigger)
   with lid
1 gallon jar
Measuring cup/spoons
Wooden spoon
Strainer
Cloth for covering jar
Rubber band to secure cloth

INGREDIENTS
1 gallon water
4 teaspoons loose tea or 4 tea
   bags (Some people brew
   with double this amount
   of tea. You can double
   this amount for a stronger
   tea flavor.)
1 cup sugar
Kombucha SCOBY
1 cup strong (vinegary)
   kombucha from
   previous batch

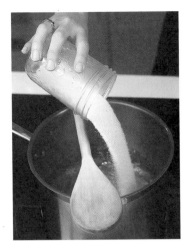

▲ Adding organic sugar to water to brew kombucha. CHRIS MCLAUGHLIN

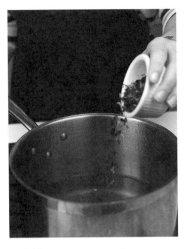

▲ Adding tea to sugar water to steep for making kombucha. CHRIS MCLAUGHLIN

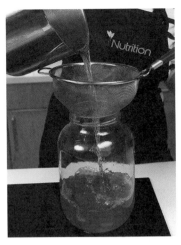

▲ Straining tea leaves and herbs into the one-gallon fermentation jar. CHRIS MCLAUGHLIN

Q: Does using metal utensils hurt the SCOBY?

A: While the kombucha and SCOBY should not have prolonged contact with metal, brief contact with stainless steel utensils will not affect the SCOBY or the kombucha. While the SCOBY and fermenting kombucha create an acidic environment, brief contact with metal funnels, strainers, stirring utensils, or tongs is not enough for a chemical reaction resulting in corrosion. Commercial kombucha brewing is actually done in stainless steel vats, just like wine. But only very high-grade stainless steel is safe for fermenting kombucha, so for homebrewers, stick to food-grade glass jars.

Directions

Making the Tea

1. Always start with clean equipment.
2. Boil water and sugar in a pot, stirring to dissolve sugar.
3. Lift the pot off the hot burner, add your tea to steep, and cover with a lid.

4. Let steep for 3–10 minutes, according to how strong you want the tea.

5. Strain tea through a sieve or tea strainer into the glass jar in which you will be fermenting the kombucha.

   WARNING Be sure that this container is meant to withstand hot liquid so it will not shatter. If you're not sure, strain into another pot or take the tea bags out and let cool before transferring it to the fermenting jar.

6. Let cool completely. The kombucha can be blood temperature or cooler, but never hot.

Fermenting (Primary Fermentation):

1. Add the SCOBY and the strong kombucha to the cooled tea.

2. Cover with a clean cloth and put in a room-temperature place, leaving it undisturbed during fermentation. Do not place directly in the sun, but a countertop or pantry shelf is fine.

3. During this time, you may notice a clear or whitish film developing on the surface. Don't be alarmed—this is the new SCOBY forming. Sometimes the Mother is attached to the Baby, but not necessarily. This "Baby" kombucha will become thicker the longer you leave it to ferment.

4. Sometimes the SCOBY sinks right when you add it to the tea, other times it floats right away. If it sinks, watch it for a few days; it should start floating, or at least part of it will reach up to the surface of the brew, where it will start forming another SCOBY. If it sinks and does not move, it is not a viable SCOBY. Start again with a fresh one in a new batch of tea.

5. You will see brownish strands or globs floating around in the kombucha, just like you would see in unpasteurized apple cider vinegar. Some people like to drink them and others prefer to strain them out.

6. When the kombucha is done is a matter of preference. Some people like it almost like vinegar; others prefer it younger and sweeter. Most people prefer the kombucha at least six days fermented in the

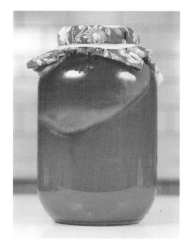

▲ SCOBY suspended in black tea kombucha. CHRIS MCLAUGHLIN

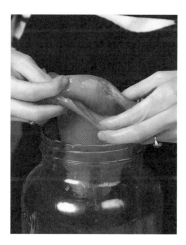

▲ SCOBY formation: the original SCOBY is on the bottom, attached to the new growth. CHRIS MCLAUGHLIN

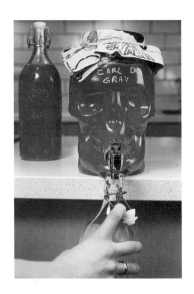

▲ Decanting with a spigoted jar makes bottling easy. CHRIS MCLAUGHLIN

primary fermentation, resulting in a tangy, but still slightly sweet kombucha. Some people brew it for up to two weeks or even longer.

The best way to know when it is done is to push the forming SCOBY aside and taste some, using a straw. It should taste at least slightly acidic. It may have a bit of effervescence. You can drink the kombucha, plain, just as it is, with little to no carbonation. Or you may choose to add more fizz and fun flavors by doing a secondary fermentation. Is it *done* yet?! Once your kombucha tastes slightly to very acidic (according to your preference), you can enjoy it as is, straight from the jar. Once you're removed the SCOBY, you can drink it plain without even bottling it or adding any additional flavors. If you don't prefer a very carbonated drink, this may be how you prefer it. Enjoy! If you want to add more fizz and some different flavors, continue onto the secondary fermentation and bottling step.

7. Once done to your taste, just remove the original and the newly forming SCOBYs from the jar (using your clean hand, a wooden spoon, or plastic or metal tongs), placing them in a clean jar, adding at least 1 cup or enough of the kombucha from this batch to cover the SCOBYs. Place a cloth cover over the jar to prevent fruit flies from entering. This jar is now your SCOBY Hotel. If you are not ready to brew another batch right away, see pages 51–52 for how to store your SCOBYs until your next batch.

Secondary Fermentation and Bottling: Adding Fizz and Flavor (Optional):

Although the SCOBY is no longer floating around in the tea, it has imparted the tea with plenty of its yeast and bacteria. Now that the SCOBY is removed from the kombucha, adding a bit more sugar will result in another round of feeding for the friendly kombucha microbes, resulting in more carbonation and some fun flavors.

NOTE By fermenting added sugar in the bottle, alcohol content also increases—by up to 2–2.5 percent. This step is optional.

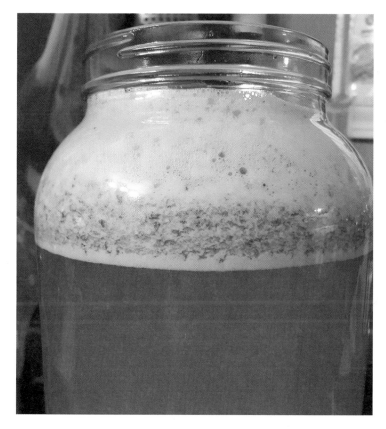

▲ Strawberries and tarragon are blended and added to kombucha before bottling and secondary fermentation, causing instant carbonation.

Secondary fermentation occurs in the bottle, so get ready for this step by cleaning your bottles and funnel or siphon.

Adding Flavor and Carbonation to Your Batch

Method 1: Flavor the Whole Batch

You can flavor the whole batch, stirring the ingredients into the gallon jar that you fermented in, and then promptly bottling to contain the fizz. This method results in even distribution of the secondary flavor, resulting in more even carbonation in the bottles. Juices, syrups and purees work best for this method.

The chart here is the Method 1 way of secondary fermentation, to flavor a whole gallon batch.

If I plan to flavor a batch, I usually stick to a neutral flavor for the primary, or something that might compliment the secondary flavor. Green or black tea as a base is my go-to, but sometimes I might change it up and do hibiscus in the primary fermentation and pair it with ginger or apple in the secondary.

Once SCOBY is removed...

BATCH FLAVORING METHOD		
SECONDARY FERMENTATION INGREDIENTS	MEASUREMENTS FOR 1 GALLON (4L) BATCH	METHOD
Strawberry Tarragon	1 cup strawberries (fresh or frozen) + 5 sprigs of tarragon	Add fresh fruit and herb to the blender, adding enough kombucha to blend, stir puree into gallon batch and bottle right away.
Pomegranate Molasses	¼ cup pomegranate molasses	Add directly to gallon batch of kombucha, stirring and bottling right away.
Blackberry Basil	1 cup blackberries (fresh or frozen) + 4 big leaves of basil	Add fresh fruit and herb to the blender, adding enough kombucha to blend, stir puree into gallon batch and bottle right away.
Mango Lassi	1 cup mango pieces (fresh or frozen) + 1 Tbsp green cardamom pods	Add fresh fruit and spice to the blender, adding enough kombucha to blend, strain puree into gallon batch and bottle right away.
Honeydew Melon	½ of a honeydew melon, skin and seeds removed, chopped into pieces	Add to blender to puree. Pour pureed pulp into gallon batch and bottle. Strain pulp when serving if desired.

Method 2: Create Different Flavors in Each Bottle

Giving each bottle a different flavor is a great way to experiment and to add variety in each batch. You can add pieces of fruit, whole sprigs of herbs, such as fresh mint, or beautiful and delicate flavors such as a piece of vanilla pod to your bottles directly, pouring the kombucha in with the flavors you choose and capping the bottles. The tricky part about this method is getting the bottles clean once you've enjoyed the kombucha from it. Some brands of store-bought kombucha have wider mouths, and reusing those bottles makes for easier cleaning than the narrow-necked beer-style bottles. You can also add syrups, fruit juices, and purees just to the bottles themselves instead of to the whole batch. How much to add is up to you, but bear in mind the sugar content of the flavoring ingredient. A syrup is very concentrated, and so start with about 1 tablespoon per 12-ounce bottle.

Secondary fermentation times vary depending on sugar content and ambient temperature. The average is 1–5 days.

The chart here is for the Method 2 way of secondary fermentation, to flavor a 1-quart bottle.

PICK-A-BERRY+HERB	About ¼ cup of your favourite berry (chopped if needed to fit in the bottle) plus a few leaves of a herb that tastes nice with it. Consider mint, basil, lemon balm, rosemary . . .
Ginger-Lemon	Chop ginger into thin slivers, adding a few to each bottle, add juice of ½ a lemon
Cinnamon-Raisin	3 Tbsp raisins + ½ a cinnamon stick (strain before drinking to enjoy!)
Mojito	Add 1 sprig of fresh mint and the juice of ½ a lime to each bottle
Blueberry-Ginger	Add a handful of blueberries and 3 thin slices of ginger (sliced into sticks so that they can get out of the bottle!)

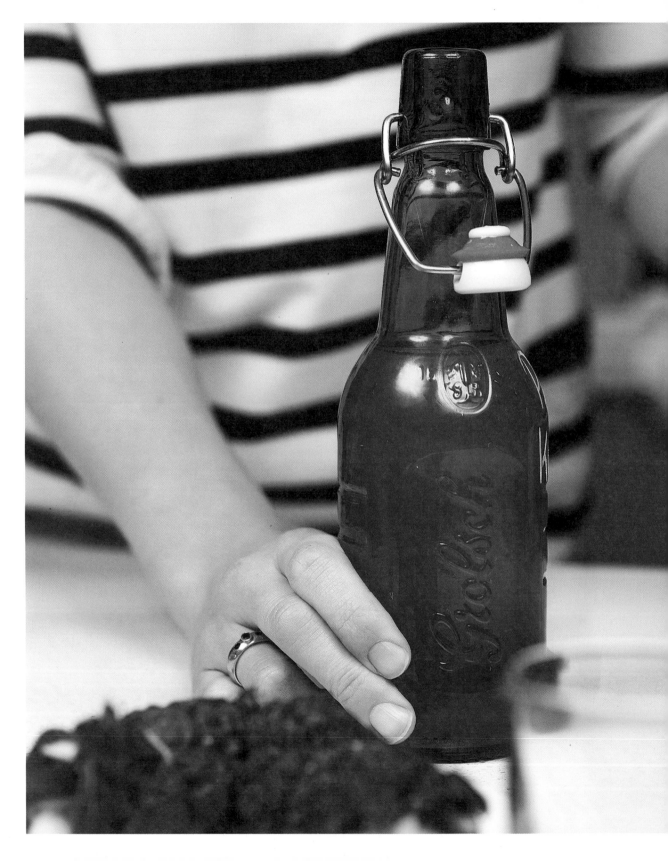

TIP Fill bottles to halfway up the neck of the bottle. Any less and there's an increased risk of overcarbonation (aka exploding bottles), too full, you won't get much fizz at all.

WARNING Adding too much additional sugar or fermenting for too long in the bottle in warm temperatures can cause overcarbonation, resulting in a sticky mess on your ceiling when you open the bottle, or even shattering the bottle.

Leaving the bottles at room temperature for at least a couple of days allows the secondary fermentation to take place. Each ingredient will have a different "fizz factor." Pureed fruit and pure fruit juices will carbonate faster than adding whole pieces of fruit. Some fruits, such fresh pineapple, are valued for their ability to add lots of carbonation.

"Burping" your bottles during secondary fermentation is advisable to avoid over- or undercarbonation. Gently releasing the pressure from the bottles allows you to feel and hear how much carbonation is in each bottle. Once you have satisfactory carbonation, put the bottles in the fridge where carbonation will slow down.

Avoid making an explosive! Don't forget to burp your bottles.

Q: How long does kombucha last for? Does it go bad?
A: Kombucha is acidic, and so it is essentially preserved. It will continue to ferment, even in the fridge, resulting in kombucha vinegar eventually. When brewed properly and put into clean bottles, it does not go "bad," but it might develop more acidity than you prefer.

CARE FOR YOUR MOTHER: THE SCOBY HOTEL

Kombucha is a very resilient culture, and unlike water kefir or some other cultures, the kombucha SCOBY thrives in an acidic environment and does not require much special care or feeding.

When your kombucha Mother is not actively fermenting a batch, just store her in some liquid from the previous batch in a jar, covered

◀ Be sure to fill bottles to halfway up the neck to reduce overcarbonation. CHRIS MCLAUGHLIN

with cloth, and at room temperature. You can add numerous SCOBYs to this jar, always topping up with liquid to cover them.

Maintaining the Hotel

Occasional cleaning of the hotel keeps the balance of yeasts and bacteria in check. If you see a lot of the brownish yeast strands in the hotel, it is time to clean it. To do this, just clean another jar and take each SCOBY out, discarding the excess brown strands. Do not wash the SCOBY under water, just slough off the excess yeast, add to a clean jar, and strain the kombucha liquid from the old hotel back over top of the SCOBYs. (Alternatively, add freshly fermented, strong kombucha and discard the old liquid.) Doing this once every few months, and alternating SCOBYs from the hotel to use for brewing from time to time results in strong and healthy SCOBYs and tasty kombucha.

How do you know if the SCOBY is still "good"? The only way that I know is to test it out by putting the culture into a new batch and see if it ferments. The SCOBY should float within a couple of days, or it might half float. So long as part of the original SCOBY reaches to the top of the jar, it should form a new one. You can add more than one Mother to a jar and it will ferment at about the same rate as if you only add one. If you do add more than one mother, they may grow together to form one very thick SCOBY—a Supermother.

WHAT TO DO WITH OVER-FERMENTED (VINEGARY) KOMBUCHA

Don't dump it! If a batch is too sour for everyday enjoyment, you can use the vinegary kombucha in several creative ways.

WARNING While vinegary kombucha may be used as vinegar in most applications, do not use it for canning. The pH is not the same as white vinegar. Canning requires very low (acidic) pH for safe food preservation.

▶ A SCOBY Hotel is a low-maintenance way to store SCOBYs between batches. CHRIS MCLAUGHLIN

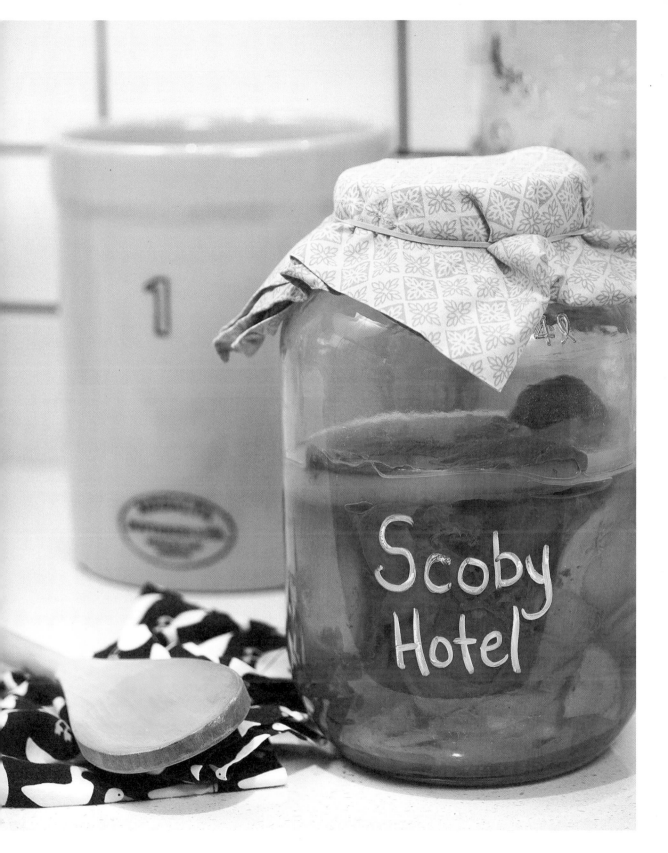

- Drink it, it's good for you! Mix it with a bit more fruit juice and drink up.
- Use it as vinegar in your favorite dressings and marinades for a promicrobial kick.
- Just as with apple cider vinegar, it can be used as an eco-friendly cleaning agent.
- Save it as starter kombucha for your next batch. Very sour kombucha will kick-start your next batch, with great results.
- Add the overfermented kombucha to your SCOBY hotel. The cultures thrive in an acidic environment.

WHAT TO DO WITH EXTRA SCOBYS

Now that you have been brewing for a while and you have given away many healthy SCOBYs to friends and family, what to do with the excess SCOBYs? Here are a few ideas.

- Your compost loves them! They tend to keep the summer stink down in your garden compost. Worms love them too. Make your worm compost happy by treating them to the occasional SCOBY.
- I have heard of chickens really enjoying them. The result seems to be eggs with thicker shells.
- Some people feed the extra SCOBYs to their pets. Dehydrated SCOBY can be a good dog chew toy. Be warned—there is hot debate among pet owners as to whether this practice is wise. Caffeine is toxic to dogs, so residual caffeine in your kombucha may harm your pup. Try brewing with the noncaffeinated herbs if you want to go for this option.
- Eat them?! Okay, I will leave this up to your experimentation. Some people are slicing and dicing, dehydrating, frying, and marinating their SCOBYs to make fruit leather, vegan jerky, squid-like sashimi and more. SCOBYs are basically cellulose (housing a wide array of bacteria and yeast strains). Humans cannot digest cellulose; we lack the enzymes needed to do so. So what's the point? Well, it's a novel use of what might be thrown out, and also, since cellulose is

not digested, it is fiber that passes through the digestive tract, potentially contributing to better intestinal tone, a cleaner digestive tract and better formed stools.

- There actually is a market for them. Try joining a buy/sell/trade site and see if you can trade that healthy SCOBY for something you need, such as some organic tea perhaps.

KOMBUCHA AND
SCOBY TROUBLESHOOTING

SCOBY sinks to the bottom of your fermentation vessel It is likely not viable. To be sure, make a batch and wait a couple of days. If no part of it floats and it is not forming any new SCOBY on top, it is best to start with a fresh SCOBY.

SCOBY is not growing very thick While it is reassuring to see nice, thick SCOBY growth, it is possible that the SCOBY can make healthy and tasty batches with minimal actual growth itself. Under some conditions it will grow thicker, but I put less weight into the importance of growing a beautiful SCOBY, and more into whether the kombucha it brews shows the signs of fermentation and tastes good.

Kombucha is not fizzy Remember that yeast is responsible for carbonation. Under warmer conditions the SCOBY will have more active yeast, so if fermentation temperature is too cool, you will get less fizz. Some people set their fermenting kombucha onto a warming mat or even knit the jar a sweater. Crafty kombucha brewers! Also, refer to carbonation section in Chapter 1.

Kombucha is too sour The sourness of kombucha is the work of acid-producing bacteria. The longer a batch ferments, the more sour it tastes (and the less sugar it contains). Try fermenting for less time next time, and either enjoy your sour kombucha mixed with fruit juice, or use in the kitchen as vinegar.

Another reason for too sour kombucha is too much SCOBY-to-liquid ratio. If the SCOBYs are too thick or numerous, thin them out by moving them to the SCOBY Hotel or composting extras. A gallon batch only needs one SCOBY, about the size of a smallish pancake, to ferment a batch.

Sediment Some batches can create quite a bit of sediment. In beer- and winemaking we call this *lees*. This sediment is spent yeast from the brewing process. It is also high in B vitamins, so I suggest you stir it in when you are bottling the kombucha.

White spots on kombucha SCOBY or floating on top of kombucha: Check very carefully. White bubbles can gather and look like mold. If they are bubbles, no need to do anything. If they are fuzzy, see "mold" below for more.

Black spots on kombucha SCOBY Check very carefully, small pieces of tea leaves or herbs that were not strained out can look like mold. If they are just leaves or herbs no need to do anything. If they are fuzzy or seem to be anything other than leaves or tea, see "mold" below for more.

Scoby is moldy This is rare, and happens when the culture is weak. If there are fuzzy white or green spots or patches or black dots, throw it out! Do not attempt to salvage a moldy SCOBY. If not sure, do an internet images search on "moldy kombucha culture." It might be moldy if it is not used to brew often enough; if it is fed the wrong type of sugar, or not enough sugar; if batches were made without any starter liquid. If this happens, or even if you are not 100 percent sure it's *not* mold, toss the SCOBY and the kombucha it is brewing and start fresh with a new SCOBY, sanitizing all of your equipment.

Kahm yeast formation A type of yeast that is common on sauerkraut and other ferments may contaminate kombucha, especially if they are fermented in close proximity to each other. Kahm yeast is white, with a wrinkly pattern. It starts as a thin white film, and develops into a thicker yeasty blanket on top of the SCOBY or kombucha liquid. While not harmful, this yeast is an indication that the batch was contaminated, and is unwanted in kombucha. Start with a fresh SCOBY.

Brown strands or blobs These are normal parts of the culture. They can be strained out or consumed. Some SCOBYs produce a lot of them, and if you find that the kombucha tastes too yeasty, simply clean the SCOBY by pulling them away with your fingers and discard these excess yeasty strands.

SCOBY forming in bottle Kombucha culture is so strong that it will form a new SCOBY from invisible yeast and bacteria that pass through the sieve, so sometimes a SCOBY starts to form in the bottle, especially if it is left at comfortable fermenting temperatures for awhile. This is fine and normal; an indication that the batch is alive! Some folks strain them out, some gulp them down.

KOMBUCHA AS AN INGREDIENT

Although I love drinking kombucha as a straight-up refreshing drink or just over ice, something fancier is sometimes very special. Janice is a colleague of mine and I credit her with this fancy cocktail. She makes it with lots of variations based on what's seasonal and fresh. She hosts kombucha-making parties, and even offers the option to add gin to her cocktail. She mentions that this is a great introduction to kombucha for sceptics or newbies. Check out www.mahhealth.com.

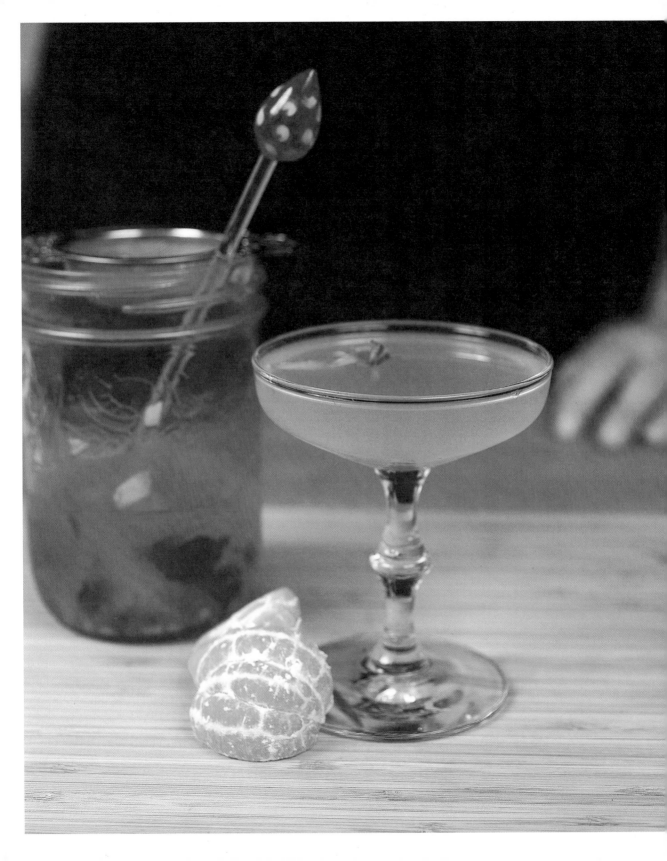

MAH'S ORANGE MINT
KOMBUCHA SPRITZ

Choose a sturdy mixing glass. Place the mint leaves into the bottom of the glass. Add orange sections. Press down lightly on the leaves and orange with muddler and give a few gentle twists. You are done when juice has released from the flesh of the orange and it smells minty. Add ice cubes and stir. Top with kombucha and strain into a beautiful glass. Serve immediately. Garnish with mint leaf.

◄ A creative ingredient in mixology: orange and mint kombucha spritzer.
CHRIS MCLAUGHLIN

Serves 2

5–8 mint leaves

1–2 mandarin oranges

¾ cup green tea kombucha— (Janice suggests cherry ginger flavored)

2 ounces gin (optional)

5–6 medium sized ice cubes

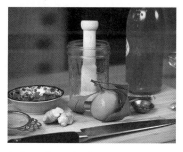

▲ Ingredients for Orange-mint Kombucha cocktail. CHRIS MCLAUGHLIN

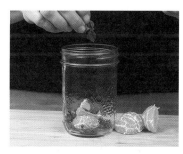

▲ Add fresh fruit and mint.
CHRIS MCLAUGHLIN

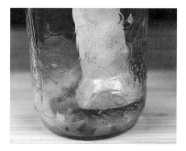

▲ Muddling ingredients for kombucha cocktail. CHRIS MCLAUGHLIN

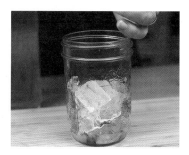

▲ Adding ice to kombucha cocktail. CHRIS MCLAUGHLIN

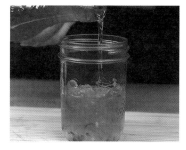

▲ Adding cherry-ginger flavored kombucha to the cocktail. CHRIS MCLAUGHLIN

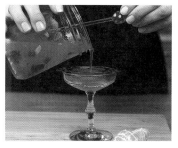

▲ Pouring the virgin kombucha cocktail. CHRIS MCLAUGHLIN

COCONUT KEFIR
KOMBUCHA SMOOTHIE

Makes 1 big smoothie

1 banana

½ cup frozen berries or
frozen cherries

⅓–½ cup coconut kefir (see
recipe on page 83). You can
substitute dairy kefir
or plain yogurt.

Kombucha—any flavor, but
I recommend a plain
green tea or berry-
flavored kombucha.

1. Add banana, berries, and coconut kefir to blender and add kombucha fill up to the 8-ounce mark on your blender.

2. Blend until smooth.

3. Keep in mind that this smoothie is lively! If you put it in a jar or bottle and carry it with you, be prepared for a bit of a carbonated burp when you open the vessel.

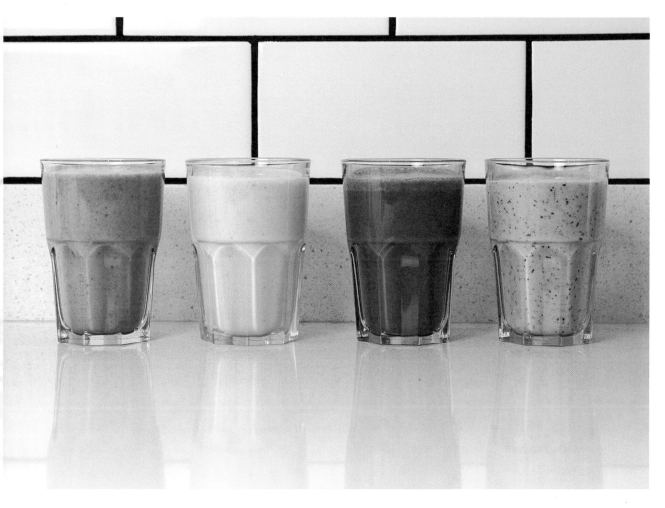

▲ Kombucha smoothies: beet berry, turmeric, spirulina, and blueberry.

CHRIS MCLAUGHLIN

3

JUN
THE HONEY-LOVING
SCOBY

JUN (**PRONOUNCED TO** rhyme with *nun* or *noon* depending on who you ask) is a relative of kombucha, but adapted to eat honey instead of sugar. It is generally more rare to find than kombucha (both the SCOBY as well as the brewed drink), for reasons you'll see below, but it is having an uprising of popularity now. Jun has an air of mysticism around it—it is said to be the stuff that Tibetan monks drank to stay alert during morning meditation. There does not seem to be any mention of Jun in ancient Tibetan texts, so perhaps it was a well-kept secret, although some think that the Jun SCOBY is a more modern genetic version of kombucha, adapted to prefer honey over sugar.

Jun first came into my world when my friend, Cierra, started brewing it. Cierra was one of my earliest fermentation workshop students. She became, first, an avid brewer of kombucha—with half a dozen flavors available to friends and housemates at all times, their brew setup was glorious! On one visit to their community house, I saw various jars with SCOBYs floating in them, each jar covered in writing. As words of positivity guarded and infused the kombucha, each jar was being imbued with intention and good vibes. This was the perfect home for Jun, one that takes great care and brings intention to the brewing process.

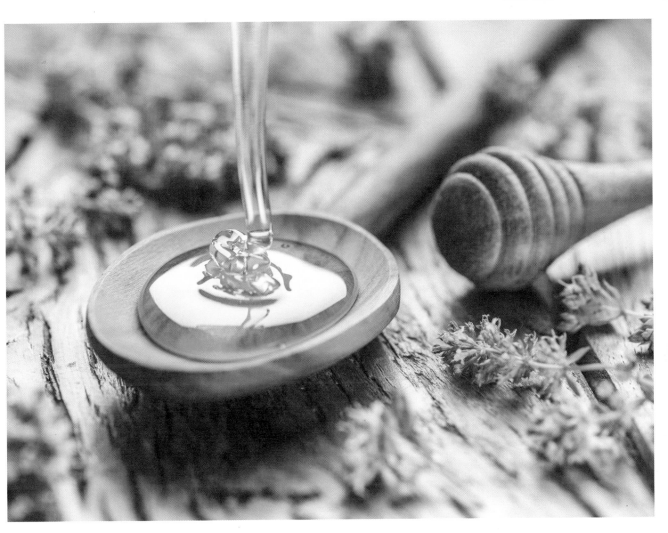

▲ Honey for making Jun should be unpasteurized and, ideally, raw. ISTOCK

Many years later, Cierra has brought her love of Jun to the world. She cofounded a business called Unity Jun, that distributes their rainbow-hued, sparking elixirs locally on Vancouver Island. Her title is "Captain and Brew Mother of Unity Jun." I love it!

I obtained a Jun SCOBY from Cierra's lineage and brewed for a while. It is truly a beautifully clean and lovely drink. But compared to kombucha, it is quite "sensitive," and due to its taste for local, raw honey, it is also more expensive to make. I have found that the

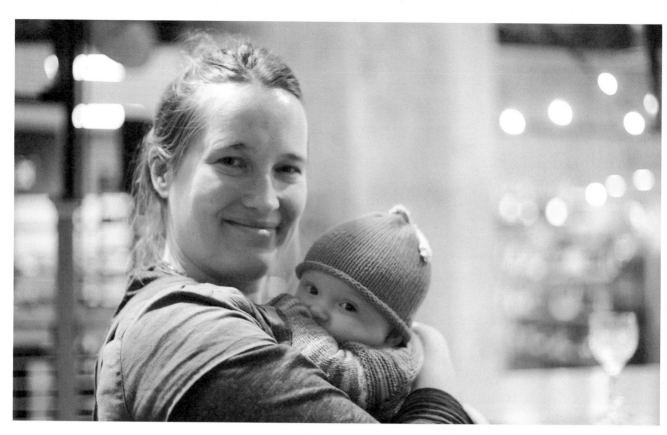

▲ Cierra, with her baby, Lucia, selling Jun at a local market. UNITY JUN

rhythm that Jun prefers does not fit well into my weekly projects schedule, so I have left the brewing of Jun to folk who can really give it the care and attention that it needs to thrive.

Since I have not perpetuated the Jun SCOBY, and they truly are tricky to track down (at least in my part of the world), I was thrilled to find out that Unity Jun will ship a "SCOBY Love Package" anywhere in the world, including a detailed recipe book and care instructions, the same organic green tea that she uses, a healthy Jun SCOBY, and even a 1 gallon jar to get started.

I caught up with Cierra to ask more about Jun.

Jun showed up in Cierra's life when her new housemate came up from California with some of the elixir and an inspired idea to start a Jun company. The concept of a kombucha-like drink that ate honey instead of sugar thrilled Cierra, as she has a self-described obsession with bees. She was on board immediately, and the friendship and business partnership was formed.

She describes the taste of Jun as more delicate than kombucha, sweeter and lighter. It is sometimes described as "the champagne of kombuchas." She surmises that because honey is a more complex sugar than cane sugar, Jun has a more diverse flavor profile, due to more diverse bacterial activity in the fermentation.

The Jun SCOBY looks physically less firm and more gooey and gloopy than the kombucha SCOBY. By maintaining any microbial culture, you get to know the character of that particular strain. Its quirks and preferences are reflected in how vigorously fermentation happens and, in the case of SCOBYs, how strong the culture itself looks. When I asked Cierra about the personality of the Jun SCOBY, she describes it as "a higher maintenance companion" than the kombucha SCOBY.

She has noticed that Jun is more sensitive to energetic vibration, temperature, and physical location. It does not like being moved once it finds a comfortable brewing zone, and prefers a cooler temperature than kombucha. Cierra notes that Jun can also be thrown off by mediocre ingredients and prefers high quality inputs. By this, she means that Jun is a real tea connoisseur. Always use organic and whole leaf green tea.

The honey she uses is raw and preferably local. She would never heat the honey (as I have seen in some recipes), preferring to brew the tea first, cool it, and add the honey once the tea is cooled, so that it keeps its own health-enhancing qualities and has more to offer the SCOBY in terms of nutrients.

Unity Jun also uses some very special water. If you come into contact with Unity Jun, I encourage you to ask them about the story of their sacred water. In the Jun lab, they use water that has undergone reverse osmosis (always use purified water for Jun) and they add a drop of water which has been collected from all parts of the globe and made sacred by being blessed in ceremony under a full moon and much more. ("Some real hippy stuff," Cierra noted.) It seems that the process Cierra uses to brew the Jun really honors the mystical lineage of the culture.

They infuse nutritional and medicinal herbs into their various elixirs. Cierra's favorite is also mine: The Om Eye Goddess flavor which uses lavender, tulsi (holy basil), and rose in addition to the green tea. Not only is it divinely tasty, Cierra notes that is fun to make because when you add the rose petals, it turns pink almost immediately.

You can get Jun SCOBY Love Package (culture) at www.unity jun.com.

There are a few key differences between care and brewing for kombucha and Jun.

For one thing, Jun prefers a cooler brewing temperature. If you have a cooler space in your home, try brewing there. If not, your Jun might just take less time to brew than the indicated times. You'll know it was too warm or too long a fermentation time if your Jun is very sour.

REMEMBER Do not heat the honey!

Kombucha is pretty forgiving when it comes to adding different flavors in the primary fermentation, such as flavored teas, alternative herbs, etc., whereas Jun requires a stricter diet of just green tea. You can still make tasty flavored Jun, but do this in the secondary fermentation so that the SCOBY is not affected.

The quality of the water seems to matter more with Jun than with kombucha. Use purified water. Likewise, the quality of tea is more important, so always use organic, preferably loose leaf (but organic bagged tea can work too).

Do not disturb the Jun during brewing except to gently push the SCOBY back under the liquid if it starts to grow up the sides of the jar.

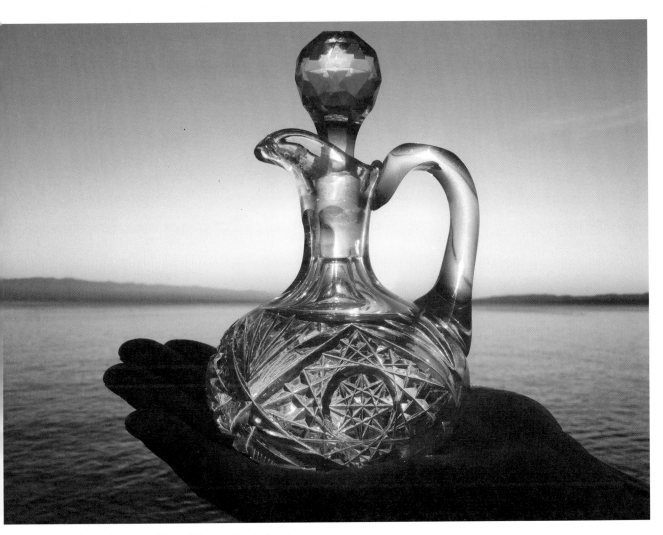

▲ Imbuing the water with good vibes makes the best Jun. UNITY JUN

Jun can be much fizzier than kombucha, so do not let the closed bottles sit at room temperature for too long. Refrigerate the Jun once the fizz factor is to your liking, and drink it fresh.

The alcohol can be higher than for kombucha—more than 2 percent. (But the stuff that Cierra sells with Unity Jun is assured to be under 0.5 percent.)

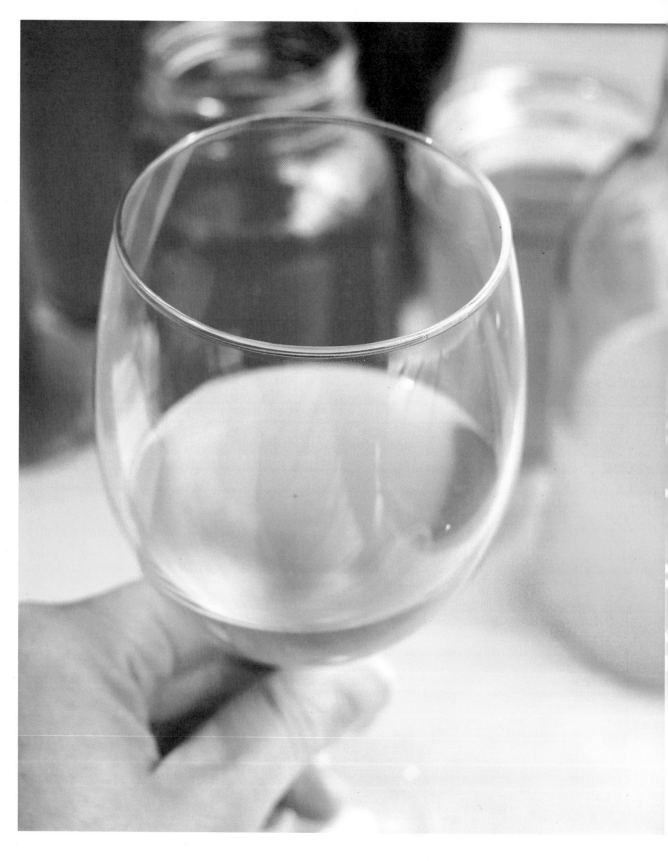

This recipe is what I use to brew, and many homebrewers use similar ratios of honey and tea to water. The process to making great Jun starts with brewing a good batch of tea. Since the expense of the ingredients may be a factor, I encourage you to use a log book, or mark your calendar to make sure that you remember when you brewed, and when to remove the SCOBY so that the tea does not over-sour.

Directions

Making the Tea

1. Boil water and add tea, putting a lid on the pot as the tea infuses for 3–5 minutes before straining the tea into the brewing jar. (Longer brewing times bring out the tannins in the tea, making a more bitter taste.)
2. Cool the tea to room temperature and stir honey in until dissolved.

Fermenting (Primary Fermentation)

1. Add the Jun SCOBY along with the cup of brewed Jun starter tea from a previous batch.
2. Jun prefers to ferment on the chillier side of room temperature. Put in a cool place to ferment, undisturbed, for around 1 week. I have fermented Jun at regular room temperature, alongside my kombucha. I find it may take a day less time to brew if it's at warmer temperatures.
3. After the initial week or so, you can dip in to taste the brew. It should be slightly acidic and may or may not already be effervescent. If it is still very sweet, you may want to leave it for another day. Once the sourness is to your liking, you can drink the Jun just as it is, removing the SCOBY.

> Makes 1 gallon (4L)
> Time: 10–15 minutes prep
>   (plus cooling time)
> Fermentation: around 1 week
>
> **EQUIPMENT**
> Pot (1 gallon or bigger)
>   with lid
> 1 gallon jar
> Measuring cup/spoons
> Wooden spoon
> Strainer
> Cloth for covering jar
> Rubber band to secure cloth
>
> **INGREDIENTS**
> 4 quarts (4L) purified water
> 4 teaspoons of loose leaf,
>   organic green tea (or 4
>   organic green tea bags)
> 1 cup raw honey
> Jun SCOBY with 1 cup of
>   Jun from previous batch

◀ Jun which has infused with Butterfly Pea Flowers in addition to green tea for vibrant color.

Optional Secondary Fermentation

Most people prefer a fizzier drink, perhaps with additional flavorings. Just as with kombucha, you can add additional flavors in the secondary fermentation upon bottling. I encourage you to get creative with the flavors you add. As noted above, Jun can become very fizzy. So take precautions when opening the bottles, and refrigerate the bottled Jun once it becomes carbonated. You can somewhat control the excess carbonation as well as alcohol production by either not adding sugary fruits or syrups to the secondary, opting instead for herbs without sugar such as fresh mint or a vanilla bean.

Care for the Jun SCOBY

The same recommendation goes for Jun as for Kombucha—just keep them separate from each other if you are keeping both. I recommend a SCOBY hotel—that is, keep excess SCOBYs in a jar, covered in plenty of Jun brewed from previous batches. Cover the jar with a tightly woven cloth cover. You won't need to feed the hotel or do much at all, just rotate the backup SCOBYs into your weekly brews to keep them happy.

4

WATER KEFIR

WATER KEFIR CULTURE

Ever since kombucha has exploded onto store shelves as the coolest drink in the functional beverages category (which, according to industry folks, means they have a perceived or real health benefit as their primary appeal), people have been searching for the next cool thing in drinks to commercialize. Some companies are already cracking the code, but water kefir is far from new. It lends itself best to homemade or microbrewed batches, so I think it will be a while before they get it right. In the meantime, I recommend you search out some kefir grains and try it for yourself.

Water kefir, also known as sugar kefir, fruit kefir, tibicos, and ginger beer plant, among other names, is a probiotic, fizzy drink that can range from quite sweet to very lemony. Water kefir has many variations and is used to ferment drinks in many corners of the world, from Hawaii to the Philippines and South and Central America. It has different local names, and slightly varied appearance in terms of the opacity and strength of the physical grains. The cultures passed around locally have adapted to local fruit sugars, and each carries a different complex of bacteria and yeasts.

Some people prefer it to kombucha for its clean, less-yeasty taste, which is sometimes compared to sparkling lemonade or cider. Since

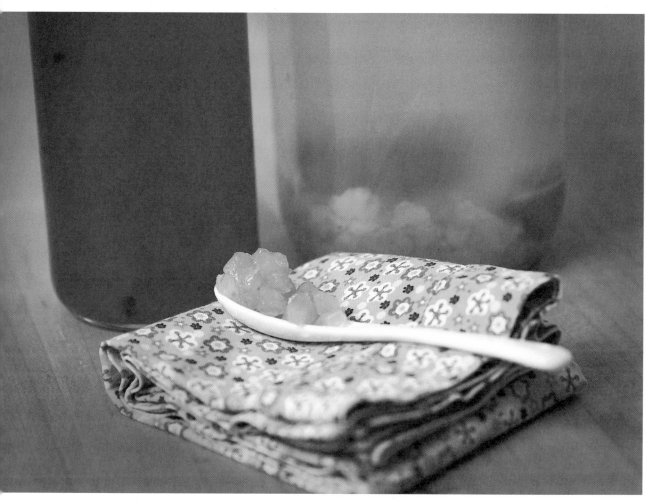

▲ Water kefir grains alongside a batch of fermenting water kefir.
CHRIS MCLAUGHLIN

no tea or herbs are necessarily added, it also does not have that slightly bitter taste that kombucha can have.

The water kefir culture is referred to as kefir grains. Quite unlike the kombucha SCOBY pellicle, and also unrelated to dairy kefir, (which looks more like gelatinous cauliflower florets), the translucent, gelatinous "grains" range in size from tiny gravel-like bits to pieces as big as marbles. They are somewhat fragile, breaking apart when stirred or handled. A matrix of live bacterial cultures, proteins, and

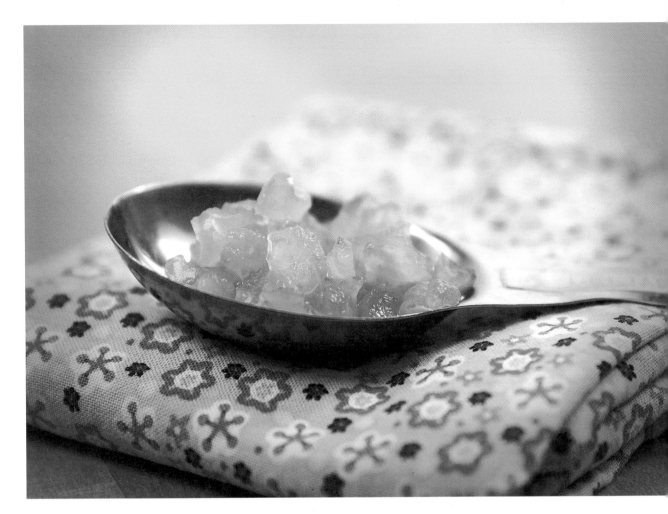

▲ The composition of water kefir grains varies slightly in appearance and texture. Some are more firm and some break up easily by stirring or shaking them. CHRIS MCLAUGHLIN

yeasts, water kefir grains are actually another form of SCOBY, different from kombucha or Jun, but a Symbiotic Culture of Bacteria and Yeast nonetheless.

WHERE TO GET WATER KEFIR GRAINS

As with kombucha SCOBYs, if you can track down a community of people who ferment various foods and drinks, you can bring up water kefir, and soon be hot on the tracks of someone who makes it and will share the grains with you. In my experience, since the grains are somewhat more care-intensive than kombucha, they are a bit trickier to track down. Labs that grow and ship cultures—Cultures for Health as well as GEM Cultures—will ship dried, live (not powdered) water kefir cultures that you can rehydrate using their instructions. They should liven back up and start brewing soon, even reproducing so you can share them with your friends.

WHAT TO FEED WATER KEFIR

The medium that water kefir grains prefer is plain sugar, along with some nutrients from fruit.

The most reliable method for fermenting water kefir is with plain, refined sugar, filtered/clean (but not distilled) water and, optionally, some pieces of fruit to flavor and add some nutrients. You can also culture coconut water or fruit juice, but I recommend always keeping some kefir grains in a sugar medium as backup.

The following recipe yields a smaller quantity than the others in this book. Because the fermentation time is short (2–5 days) and the grains need to be fed regularly, it makes sense to make smaller batches more often to keep the grains in regular use.

NOTE Unlike kombucha SCOBYs, the water kefir grains do not thrive in a very acidic medium. If you overbrew your grains, they will literally pickle. These somewhat more fragile grains need to be moved to another batch of sweetened water every two, or maximum three days to stay healthy. I overbrewed a batch once and the grains shrunk almost to the point of disappearing. Needless to say, I had to start over with fresh grains when I was ready to be a better kefir caretaker.

FERMENTING FRUIT JUICES AND ADDING SYRUPS

Kefir grains can ferment fruit sugars too, so you can experiment with your excess grains (always keep some in plain sugar water). Fruit juices that are not too acidic work to produce a fizzy drink. Just put

4–5 tablespoons of grains into pear, apple, apricot, peach, or berry juices. Ferment for two to three days and bottle, keeping bottles at room temperature for another two days, or until fizzy. For more acidic juices such as passion fruit, guava, citrus, etc., dilute the juice with ½ sugar–water mixture.

Coconut water kefir has a loyal following among health-motivated fermenters. The idea is that it combines the enzyme and probiotic qualities of water kefir with the electrolyte properties of coconut water (not to be confused with coconut milk). After having tried this, I can wholeheartedly say that I am *not* among that loyal following. After the natural sugars are fermented out of the coconut water, I was left with a salty-tasting, bland, and fizzy drink. I don't want to deter you from experimenting, this is just my review. If you do have access to lots of coconut water, do try it for yourself—I see potential for it as an ingredient in smoothies, etc., but I'll pass on it as a sipper in its own right.

Syrups can be added. Start with 1 tablespoon of syrup in the secondary (bottled) fermentation. Add maple syrup, molasses, pomegranate molasses, or any fruit concentrate syrup or cordial that you love.

WATER KEFIR
BASIC RECIPE

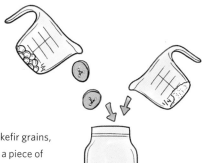

1. In a 1L jar, add active kefir grains, sugar and optionally, a piece of fresh or dried fruit.

2. Put a lid on and shake it up.

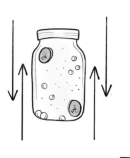

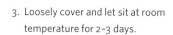

3. Loosely cover and let sit at room temperature for 2–3 days.

4. Strain out the liquid and enjoy it now.

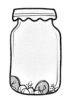

5. For more fizz, transfer to tightly sealed bottles and let sit for 2 or more days. Enjoy fresh or refrigerate.

Makes 1 quart (1L)

Time: 2 minutes prep

Fermentation: 2–5+ days

EQUIPMENT

1-quart jar with lid

Tightly woven cloth with rubber band

Strainer

Measuring cup

Bottles (recommended)

INGREDIENTS

Just under 1 quart (1L) water

¼ cup whole or refined cane sugar

4–5 tablespoons water kefir grains

Optional flavorings (see page 78). You can use whole fresh or dried fruit, flavors such as ginger or turmeric, or try adding juices or syrups to the secondary fermentation

---

▲ How to make kefir. CRYSTAL ALEXANDRIA

in the bottle instead.

You can add these flavors to the jar for the initial fermentation stage, or you can add pieces of fruit to the bottles for secondary fermentation and strain them out to serve.

Banana Surprisingly tasty and subtle, just add ¼ peeled banana. Add a slice of fresh turmeric for a pretty golden color.

Blackberry ginger Add ¼ cup blackberries plus a few slices of ginger.

Perry orchard Tastes like pear cider. Substitute apples for apple cider taste. Just add 2 or 3 slices of good eating pear or apple (with peel on).

Love potion Add 1 stalk of pink rhubarb and ¼ vanilla pod, split lengthwise.

Figgy fruitcake Add one fig, split in half, or a couple of prunes. When adding dried fruit, be sure it's unsulfured. The taste of this is very subtle, but dried fruits add some depth of flavor to the otherwise tangy spritzer type of drink.

Floral Without adding extra sugar, you can infuse your bottled water kefir with rosewater or orange blossom water, or with a sprig of lavender. I recommend adding these to the bottles once you have poured the liquid off of the grains. About 1 teaspoon: 1 quart (1L) works for the rosewater and orange blossom water, or 1 sprig of lavender.

Directions

1. The method I use for making water kefir is quick and lazy. Some methods call for boiling water, adding sugar, and cooling it. I have found that I can skip heating water and just shake the jar to dissolve the sugar. The easier I can make it, the better, as this culture needs to be fed pretty often. This method requires that you have good-quality, filtered water. Some prefer to boil the water and cool it.

2. In a clean quart jar, add sugar and water, screw the lid on tightly, and shake to dissolve sugar. Add water kefir grains (and optional fruits/flavorings as listed). Be sure to either loosen the lid or take it off, opting for a tightly woven cloth cover, secured with a rubber band instead.

3. Adding a piece of fruit or flavoring here is optional, but adds some subtle flavor and allows you to skip out on having to do a secondary flavoring later. The nutrients from the fruits can help the water kefir grains stay healthy. If you add fruit, it's easiest to keep it in large pieces, so use a good wedge of apple, a whole dried fig or prune, some

thick chunks of banana, etc. Some brewers like to keep the fruit out of the equation until secondary fermentation (once you pour the liquid off the grains) which makes for tidier-looking grains (you won't have to dig around them to get out any lemon pits or blackberry seeds).

Fermenting the Brew

Let the kefir sit at room temperature for 2–3 days. You may not notice any change during this period, but signs that fermentation has occurred are that there's a slightly acidic but fresh smell with a lemony taste and perhaps slight effervescence. The grains may have noticeably increased in volume, but also may not have; both can result in healthy and tasty water kefir.

Bottling

If you added fruit or other flavorings, skim from the top as best you can with a clean spoon. Compost or eat the fruit.

Using a sieve and funnel, strain mixture into a bottle, placing kefir grains in a clean jar, ready for next use. Cap the bottle.

Keep the bottle at room temperature for another 2 days or more. Check the fizziness by letting the pressure off the bottles, listening for that release of gas. Once you are satisfied with the fizz factor, drink right away or refrigerate for up to a few weeks.

Want to add more flavor and fizz? You can add more sugar, fruit pieces, or fruit purees to the bottle, just as with kombucha. Experiment by adding some mango puree, fruit syrup, or fresh berries to the bottle.

CARING FOR YOUR KEFIR GRAINS

Use grains for another batch immediately—this is best for growth and heath of grains. Or, you could take a break from making water kefir.

For a short break (1–3 weeks), store grains in fresh water and sugar (same proportions as when you make a batch) and store in

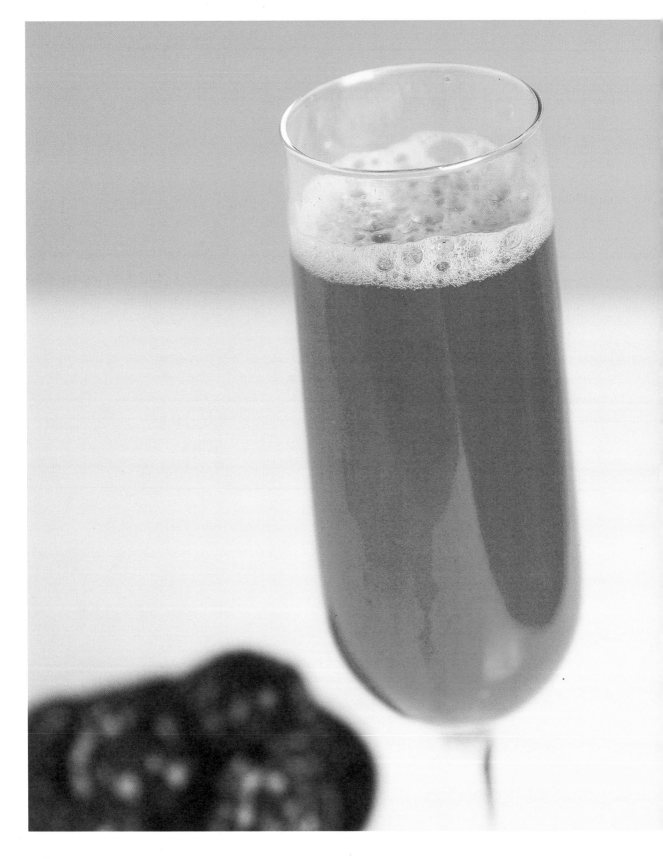

the fridge with a tight lid on. When you are ready to start brewing again, return it to room temperature. You may drink the liquid, but if it has an unpleasant smell, just pour out the liquid and start a new batch. It can sometimes take a couple of batches to get your grains happy again.

For a longer break (a few months), dry the grains. Just place them on a piece of unbleached paper towel and let them air dry for a few days. If you live in a humid climate, you may need to dehydrate the grains in a food dehydrator (no hotter than 85°F [30°C]). Once the kefir grains are dried, store them in an airtight bag in the fridge.

To bring them back to life, rehydrate them by mixing up one batch of sugar water as below. Let sit for 3 days, pour off that liquid then start brewing as usual.

REMAINING SUGAR AND ALCOHOL

The fermented water kefir has about 20 percent the amount of sugar of the original and almost all of it has been converted from sucrose to fructose. As glucose is consumed by the grains and turned into beneficial organic acids and CO_2 (fizz), and very small amounts of alcohol (usually about 0.5–0.75 percent, but can climb up to ~3 percent under the right conditions).

A RHYTHM OF ITS OWN

Water kefir takes 2–6 days to ferment, a relatively quick process. The culture is a bit more sensitive than kombucha culture. If it is left to overferment, the acid that results from the conversion of sugar can actually harm and then kill the culture. Water kefir grains prefer to be fed quite often which is why when I brew mine, I make 1 quart at a time, keeping a rotating jar of water kefir on the counter, mixing up a new batch every few days as I bottle the last batch. Once you find how much water kefir your household consumes per week, you can find your rhythm. Halve or double the batch to keep your culture fed regularly.

◀ Blackberry-flavored water kefir.
CHRIS MCLAUGHLIN

Q: Do kefir grains reproduce?

A: They can, but are sometimes hesitant to do so. So long as my kefir continues to taste fresh and ferment in a couple of days, I don't worry too much about whether the grains are reproducing. Water kefir grains can ferment successful batches indefinitely if they are cycled through batches regularly. Some folks have noticed that they reproduce better in hard water (water high in mineral content). People have been known to add clean egg shells, a pinch of baking soda, or a slice of lemon to get those water kefir grains into reproduction mode. Under some conditions, (such as ideal water minerals and pH) their population may explode; some brewers also report a seasonal boost in population in the springtime—if this is the case; just maintain each 1-quart batch with about 4–5 tablespoons of grains. With the extra grains, dry them for backup, give them to your friends, or even drink them.

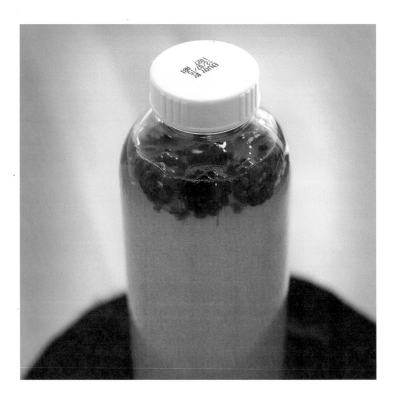

▶ Whole berries flavoring water kefir in the bottle.
CHRIS MCLAUGHLIN

COCONUT KEFIR YOGURT
RECIPE

Here's another use for your coconut water grains—a coconut kefir yogurt recipe.

I met Ellexis at a local culinary school where she was working as assistant to the pastry instructor and I showed up to instruct a guest day on healthy cooking classes. Since then, we have been enthusiastically encouraging each other's nerdy culinary and nutrition interests for years, and she is co-teaching a series of healthy cooking classes with me. She has taught me much in the ways of plant-based baking, and I have passed on my fermentation fervor to her. Her classes are all plant based, and so for her "Un-Dairy Your Kitchen" class, she developed this tangy and super-rich coconut cream/yogurt, which uses water kefir grains to get started.

Once you have started one batch with the water kefir grains, you can actually just use the coconut yogurt itself as a starter from then on.

This is an extremely simple recipe/ferment that produces a zippy probiotic drink or, when left in the fridge for a week, will thicken into a Greek-style yogurt that is fabulous on granola, as a crema on burritos or tacos, and even served with desserts. The recipe following explains how to start your first batch of kefir using water kefir grains and then continue to make subsequent batches using only 1 tablespoon of your active ferment. I find that using the thick yogurt to inoculate makes the most active and best tasting kefir/yogurt.

Makes 1 cup

Time: 24 hours

INGREDIENTS

1 13-ounce can organic full fat coconut milk

1 teaspoon Water kefir grains or 1 tablespoon fermented coconut yogurt (from previous batch)

2 teaspoons organic pure maple syrup

Directions

1. Open can of coconut milk and pour into a jar of a similar volume with a half-inch headspace once filled with liquid.

2. Mix the maple syrup and kefir grains into the coconut milk and secure jar with a tight-fitting lid.

3. Set in your cold oven with the light on overnight. By morning it will have bubbles and start to taste sour—about 12 to 24 hours.

4. Strain the yogurt to remove the water kefir grains. Return the coconut kefir to the jar and set in the refrigerator. Drink as liquid or allow it to sit in fridge for 3 days up to 1 week when it will begin to thicken into yogurt.

5. Be sure to save 1 tablespoon from your active batch of kefir or yogurt to inoculate the next batch. The more you culture the more active and tasty it will become.

Coconut
Kefir
March 5

5

WILD-FERMENTED GINGER BEER; FRUIT AND HERBAL SODAS

GINGER BEER OR GINGER ALE?

ALTHOUGH IT IS called beer, this drink is not made from grains, and is usually enjoyed as nonalcoholic (or with minimal alcohol levels). Ginger beer has its origins in brewing, using yeast and bacterial strains of cultures. In the mid-18th century, the British were brewing a spicy ginger soda using a strain of water kefir grains. (You can also make it using a ginger bug as described here). The drink has a signature cloudiness, which results from the yeast in fermentation. It was bottled in stoneware or glass bottles, corked and wired tight, and shipped across the Atlantic, where it become popular as well. Its popularity dipped as prohibition changed the drinkscape of America. The mildly alcoholic drink was replaced by a manufactured (not fermented) drink, ginger ale.

Ginger ale is a milder soda, and like other commercial sodas, is made with carbonated water and sugar, as well as artificial flavorings and sometimes artificial colors as well. The line between ginger beer and ginger ale is blurring, as manufacturers are skipping out on fermentation, which leads to more varied results (the production of alcohol can be difficult to tame).

A recent jump in the popularity of homemade sodas has led to the rise of home-carbonation machines, but real-deal, homecrafted sodas are made fizzy by fermentation, not forced carbonation, so I stick to the oldest-style soda recipes.

WHY *WILD*-FERMENTED?

Unlike the previous projects in this book, which require you to source a starter culture, ginger beer (and any fruit or herbal soda you concoct) can be fermented using wild yeast and bacteria. This culture is called a ginger bug, and is similar to the composition of a sourdough starter. It can be made fresh every time you want to make a batch, or, with very little maintenance, can be perpetuated for quicker and more consistent results in fermentation. You can also use the active ginger bug to make lots of other fizzy drinks. Fizz up your fruit juices and craft herbal and fruit sodas as well as root beer.

Why use wild (not packaged) yeast? By making a wild-fermented ginger bug rather than using commercial bread or beer/wine yeast, your brew has a broader complement of bacteria and can have a broad spectrum of enzymes for digestion. It also means that your brews will take a varied amount of time to ferment, based on how strong your wild yeast culture is. Like other cultured beverages, the sparkling soda that results is lower in sugar than in commercially produced beverages. Some or most of the sugar is consumed in the process of fermentation, depending on brewing method and fermenting time. If you want to test how much sugar remains in your brew, get a hydrometer at your local beer brewing supply store. It's an inexpensive measuring tool for sugar and alcohol in liquids. I still consider ginger beer and wild-fermented sodas to be more of a treat than some of the other fermented beverages since these drinks have more initial and residual sugar.

MAKING AND CARING FOR A GINGER BUG

The ginger bug is a resilient culture. I discovered that the ginger bug culture could be easily maintained and readily revived, ready for fermenting a new batch of soda. Once my fermentation fervor really came into full swing, my kitchen and pantry started to transform

▶ Ginger bug.

into a laboratory. Jars and crocks bubbled away on my countertop, swing-top bottles, some closed and some with airlocks bubbling away, lined my pantry shelves, sloppily handwritten labels identified the contents and date bottled so I could more or less tell which bottles might be ready to drink or needed to be stored in the fridge.

I made my first ginger bug according to Sandor Katz's book, *Wild Fermentation*. I added the active culture to a batch of ginger and lemon tea, creating my first batch of ginger beer. All went well, but I had a lot of other projects on the go, so after I guzzled the last bottle, I must have left the bottle in the pantry without washing it out. I found that bottle a year later, labeled and dated. I noticed that a neat ring of sediment had settled to the bottom, and no liquid remained. Instead of washing the bottle, I was curious—would these yeasts spring back to life if I were to feed them?

I added some cooled sweet ginger and lemon tea to the bottle, shook it up and sealed it. And to my excited surprise, those yeasts did come back to life! Within a few days at room temperature, the contents were fizzy. The resiliency of this culture astounded me—so I kept it going. I used the ginger beer from that revived batch to make another ginger bug culture, and have been perpetually using this culture for almost nine years now. I thought that if a strain of yeast and bacterial cultures is so strong as to be able to live for a year without feeding or regulation of temperature, it would make a great pet project to maintain. Although I now keep my ginger bug culture in the fridge, it is a culture that I can either feed, care for, and use to brew regularly, or that I can shove to the back of the fridge and forget about until I am ready to make another batch. I brew ginger beer and sodas more in the summer, so for months my ginger bug is content to wait for another feeding.

The fortitude of the microbial culture that I had captured impressed me. Through experiences like this one, I have started to think of myself not just as a brewer of tasty and healthy drinks and foods, but as a steward of micro-organisms. I keep a variety of

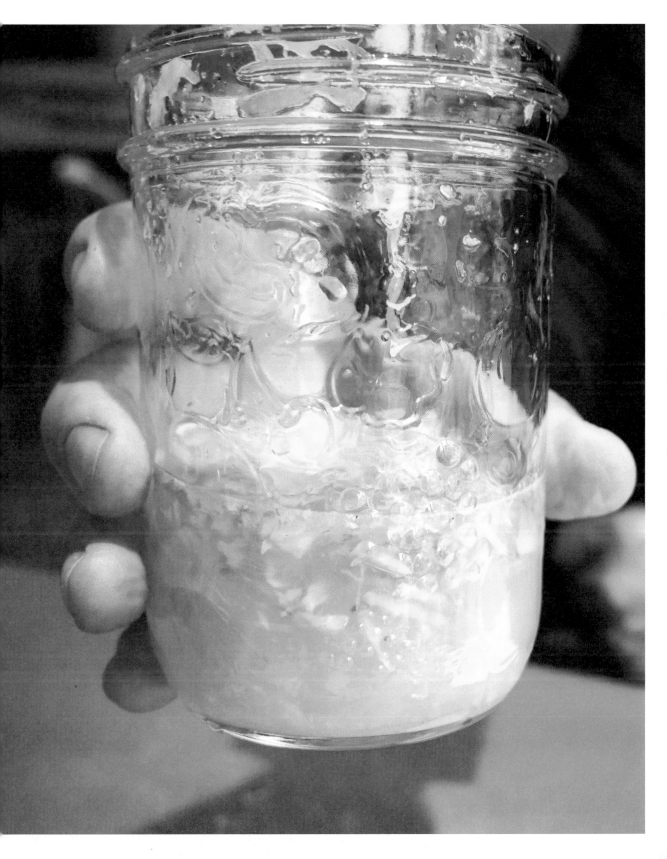

cultures alive, and by actively brewing different drinks, I contribute to a vibrant and diverse microbial community, which in turn contributes to the fortitude and resiliency of my own body systems.

Is my brew probiotic? Because ginger beer is a wild ferment, it has varied and diverse organisms, which can include beneficial bacteria. Some people add a probiotic powder to their ferment to assure probiotic activity. It's up to you if you want to culture it, or leave it up to the wild organisms. My experience is with wild organisms.

Variations and other soda flavors: Your active ginger bug can make lots of different sweet drinks into tasty, fizzy sodas. I recommend trying the basic ginger beer recipe first and then branching out to some of the other fruit and herbal sodas.

GINGER BEER
BASIC RECIPE

Makes 4 quarts (4 L)

Time: 20 minutes prep

Fermentation: 4–10 days (plus
an extra 3+ days if making
a ginger bug culture from
scratch)

EQUIPMENT

A pot with at least
4-quart capacity

Grater

Funnel

½ pint or pint jar for the
ginger bug

Measuring cups

Wooden spoon or spatula

Swing-top glass beer bottles
to 4-quart total capacity

4-quart jar or bucket

Cloth with rubber band to cover
jar or bucket (optional: if you
want to produce more alcohol)

**INGREDIENTS FOR
GINGER BUG**

⅓ cup filtered water

2 tablespoons sugar

2 tablespoons coarsely grated
organic ginger, skin on

**INGREDIENTS FOR
GINGER BEER**

¼–½ cup coarsely grated ginger,
preferably organic, packed to
measure (¼ cup makes a mild
beer and ½ cup is pretty spicy)

1½ cups sugar

Water (2 quarts + 2 quarts),
divided

2 lemons or 3 limes

Additional herbs or spices
(see page 94 for variations):
optional

Active ginger bug—about ¼ cup
strained volume

Directions

The basic process for this project and many other fermented beverages using the ginger bug as a starter is as follows

1. Make ginger bug (takes 3–10 days for first batch, but you can keep it going after this, so this is only necessary the first time you brew if you maintain the culture).
Brew a flavorful, sweetened tea and cool it down.
    Add micro-organisms (active ginger bug).
    Bottle and ferment (takes 4–10 days).
    To make the ginger bug (culture), start at least 3 days before you plan to brew (or at least 10 days before you want the brew to be completed). Grate 2 tablespoons ginger with the skin on and mix in a jar

▶ How to make Ginger Beer.

1. Make a Ginger Bug:

2. Shake everyday until bubbly.

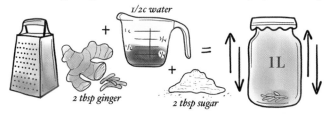

1/2c water

2 tbsp ginger

2 tbsp sugar

1L

3. Brew a strong gingery, sweetened 'tea': Add
   sugar, ginger and water to a pot and simmer.

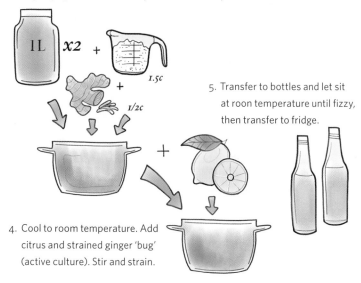

1L x2 +

1.5c

+

1/2c

5. Transfer to bottles and let sit
   at roon temperature until fizzy,
   then transfer to fridge.

4. Cool to room temperature. Add
   citrus and strained ginger 'bug'
   (active culture). Stir and strain.

with ⅓ cup water and 2 tablespoons sugar. Cover with a cloth to keep
pests out. Stir it vigorously or put a cap on to shake it at least 2 times
per day. This mixture will start to get bubbly sometime at about 2–5
days. This means that it is active and you are ready to make ginger
beer. (Congratulations—you made a ginger bug!) If you are not ready
to make a batch of soda that day, just feed it another teaspoon each
of grated ginger and sugar each day until you are ready, or put it in
the fridge, bringing it to room temperature a few hours before you
want to brew.

When You Are Ready to Make the Ginger Beer

2. **Brew a flavorful, sweetened ginger tea**
    Boil 2 quarts of water with the sugar and ginger, as well as any optional spices (like cinnamon sticks or fennel seeds). Simmer for 10 minutes.

    Once simmered, take it off of the heat and add the juice of the lemons/limes.

    Add 2 quarts cold water to cool the mixture.

    Cool the mixture to lukewarm or room temperature.

3. **Add micro-organisms (culture)**
    Add the strained ginger bug into the cooled tea and stir well. If you intend to make this an ongoing project, save a bit of your ginger bug and just feed it more ginger and sugar and top up with water. Put it in the fridge and take it out to warm up before you use it again. Make sure it's active every time you use it!

    TIP To perpetuate the ginger bug, save strained ginger bits in the jar once you have brewed a batch and poured off some of the liquid. Top up the ginger bits with a couple more tablespoons of sugar, a little more grated ginger, and enough filtered water to just cover the ginger mixture. Shake or stir to dissolve the sugar and refrigerate until you are ready to make another batch.

    On brewing day, bring the bug back up to room temperature and feed it another spoonful of grated ginger and sugar. Wait until it is nice and bubbly to add it to your cooled soda mixture. You will eventually have more volume of ginger in the bug than you need. I just toss the ginger bug into a batch of muffins (which adds flavor and lots of rising power!) or the compost.

    The ginger bug is a very low-maintenance culture; I have successfully kept mine going for years. I just store it in the fridge

between batches, sometimes for a few months without any maintenance. If your bug is having trouble getting bubbly again when you
are ready to brew, move it to a warmer place and be sure to shake it or
stir vigorously from time to time. Any sign of mold means toss it and
start again, and if you are having a difficult time getting it to restart,
just make a new one.

4. **Bottle and Ferment**

    Strain mixture into a bucket or jar.

    For nonalcoholic ginger beer, you will want to bottle it soon.
    Funnel your mixture into bottles and seal them. Let the bottles sit
    at room temperature for at least 4 days. Check the bottles daily by
    burping them, and move to the fridge when they are starting to get
    carbonated. This may take up to 10 days or so, depending on how
    active your ginger bug was when you added it. Be patient!

    NOTE If you want to make alcohol you will need to open-ferment
    this brew for a few days. Just leave it in a jar, loosely covered with a
    cloth, at room temperature. The longer you leave it, the more alcohol
    is produced. If you want to know how much alcohol is in it, purchase
    an inexpensive hydrometer from a homebrew supply store, or, alter-
    natively, you could just drink some and see how tipsy you feel. I have
    left batches in the open-fermentation stage for 10 days before bot-
    tling in order to get an adult beverage.

    ### Variations

    Lemongrass ginger beer Chop up one stalk of lemongrass and add
    it to the boil with the ginger.

    Island lower hibiscus ginger beer Add ⅓ cup hibiscus to the boil
    with the ginger.

    Digestive ginger beer Add 3 tablespoons fennel seeds and 1 cinna-
    mon stick to the boil with the ginger.

    Blueberry blush ginger beer Add 1 cup fresh or frozen blueberries
    to the boil with the ginger.

ROOT BEER

Root beer originates from the southern United States, where roots, flowers, berries, and barks would be collected and brought back to the brewmaster of the house. Sassafras, sarsaparilla, birch bark, dandelion root, juniper berries, wintergreen, and more were boiled and sorghum molasses was added. My variation here includes blackstrap molasses, which is derived from sugar cane, to give it that deep color and intensity of flavor. To make your soda fizzy, you can use an active ginger bug or water kefir grains. Whey can also be used. I recommend whey from dairy kefir or coconut milk kefir. For more on how to obtain and use whey in fermented drinks, see the Chapter 6: Whey-Fermented Drinks.

Sourcing root beer herbs is a bit of a mission. All of the herbs can be found online at Mountain Rose Herbs, which stocks a delightful variety of excellent quality herbs and spices as well as superfoods and teas.

I was excited to find the root beer mixture, already premixed at a few of my local herbal apothecaries and health food stores. It is sold as root beer tea or root beer herbs. If you avoid gluten, be sure to look at the ingredients. The premixed root beer herbs sometimes contain crystal malt, which contains gluten.

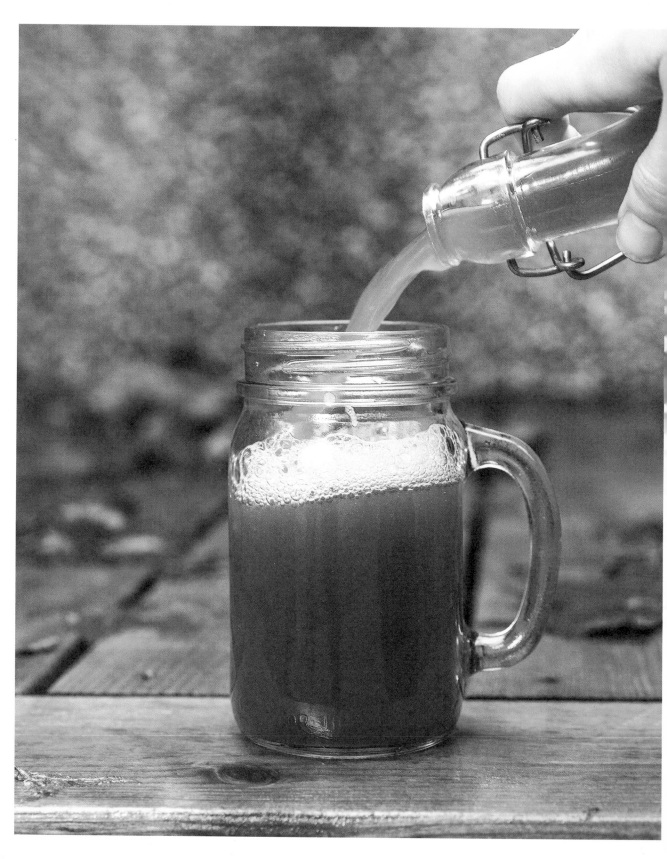

EQUIPMENT

A pot with at least 4 quarts
    (4L) capacity
Funnel
Strainer
Measuring cups
Wooden spoon or spatula
Swing-top glass beer bottles to
    4 quarts total capacity
4-quart jar or bucket
Cloth with rubber band to cover
    jar or bucket (optional: if you
    want to produce more alcohol)

INGREDIENTS

Water (2 quarts + 2 quarts)
⅓ cup root beer herbs
1¼ cups sugar
⅓ cup blackstrap unsulfured
    molasses
Culture options (choose one):
Active ginger bug: use about
    ¼ cup strained volume
Or use 1 cup whey from coconut
    kefir or dairy kefir (For more
    on how to obtain and use
    whey in fermented drinks,
    see Chapter 6.)

Or use 3–5 tablespoons water
kefir grains (spare or backup
ones—water kefir grains prefer
plain water and sugar, but can
be cycled through to make a
batch of root beer from time
to time)

Directions

1. **Brew a flavorful, sweetened root beer tea**

   Boil 2 quarts of water stirring in the sugar, root beer herbs, and
   molasses. Simmer for 20 minutes.

   Add 2 quarts cold water to cool the mixture.

   Cool the mixture to lukewarm or room temperature.

2. **Add Micro-Organisms (Culture)**

   Add the culture into the cooled tea and stir well.

   (If you are using the ginger bug and want to perpetuate it, see the
   ginger beer recipe for instructions.)

◀ Root beer fermented with ginger bug. CHRIS MCLAUGHLIN

3. **Bottle and Ferment**

Strain mixture into a bucket or jar.

For nonalcoholic root beer, you will want to bottle it soon. Funnel mixture into bottles and seal them. Let the bottles sit at room temperature for at least 4 days. Check the bottles daily by burping them, and move to the fridge when they start to get carbonated. This may take up to 10 days or so, depending which culture you used or how active your culture was when you added it. Be patient.

Variations

Root beer has many variations. Among homebrewers the recipe varied according to what was on hand and growing locally. The variation below is a more medicinal-tasting brew, but I find it to be a nicer way to take the bitter-tasting herbs that help keep my liver healthy. It's a good spring tonic.

LOVE YOUR LIVER ROOT BEER TONIC

Add ⅓ cup dandelion roots (dried) and/or ⅓ cup burdock root (dried).

I tend to brew more sodas in the summer, but this is an exception. This brew features elderberries and rosehips, which are immune-boosting herbs that can help to kick a cold. I make this during cold and flu season, but it is a tasty way to take medicine, so it would not be out of place at any time of year. Elderberries and rosehips can be found at herbal apothecaries and some health food stores, or Mountain Rose Herbs carries them so you can stock up by ordering online.

EQUIPMENT

A pot with at least 4 quarts (4 L) capacity

Funnel

Strainer

Measuring cups

Wooden spoon or spatula

Swing-top glass beer bottles to 4 quarts total capacity

4-quart jar or bucket

Cloth with rubber band to cover jar or bucket (optional: if you want to produce more alcohol)

INGREDIENTS

Water (2 quarts + 2 quarts)

1½ cups sugar

½ cup dried elderberries

½ cup dried rosehip chips or pieces

Culture options (choose one):

Active ginger bug: use about ¼ cup strained volume

Or use 1 cup whey from coconut kefir or dairy kefir

Or use 3–5 tablespoons water kefir grains (spare or backup ones—water kefir grains prefer plain water and sugar, but can be cycled through to make a batch of root beer from time to time)

Directions

1. **Brew a flavorful, sweetened elderberry and rosehip tea**

   Boil 2 quarts of water stirring in the sugar and herbs. Simmer for 10 minutes.

   Add 2 quarts cold water to cool the mixture.

   Cool the mixture to lukewarm or room temperature.

2. **Add Micro-Organisms (Culture)**

   Add the culture into the cooled tea and stir well.

   (If you are using the ginger bug and want to perpetuate it, see the ginger beer recipe for instructions.)

3. **Bottle and Ferment**

   Strain mixture into a bucket or jar.

   For nonalcoholic soda, you will want to bottle it soon. Funnel mixture into bottles and seal them. Let the bottles sit at room temperature for at least 4 days. Check the bottles daily by burping them, and move to the fridge when they start to get carbonated. This may take up to 10 days or so, depending which culture you used or how active your culture was when you added it.

TURMERIC CARDAMOM FIZZ

Turmeric is a medicinal and culinary root that gives this soda the most beautiful golden color. The earthy flavor of turmeric is balanced with the floral notes in the cardamom pods. The black pepper may seem out of place, but turmeric has a special affinity for black pepper. They are very often added together in a variety of curry dishes, and as science is catching up with traditional wisdom, we now know that black pepper works synergistically with turmeric to intensify its anti-inflammatory properties. Use fresh ginger when available; powdered is fine too. To serve, tip the bottle gently to mix the turmeric back in before pouring.

EQUIPMENT

A pot with at least 4 quarts
  (4L) capacity
Grater
Funnel
Strainer
Measuring cups
Wooden spoon or spatula
Swing-top glass beer bottles to
  4 quarts total capacity
4-quart jar or bucket
Cloth with rubber band to cover
  jar or bucket (optional: if you
  want to produce more alcohol)

INGREDIENTS

Water (2 quarts + 2 quarts)
1½ cups sugar
¼ cup fresh ginger, grated
  and packed to measure
2 "fingers" fresh turmeric
  (about 2 tablespoons
  grated) or ¾ tablespoon
  turmeric powder
10 black peppercorns
14 green cardamom pods,
  crushed
Juice of 1 lemon

Culture options (choose one):
Either ¼ cup strained volume of
  active ginger bug
Or use 1 cup whey from coconut
  kefir or dairy kefir
Or use 3–5 tablespoons water
  kefir grains (spare or backup
  ones—water kefir grains
  prefer plain water and sugar,
  but can be cycled through to
  make a batch of root beer
  from time to time)

Directions

▶ Tumeric cardamom soda made with ginger bug. HONAMI WATANABI

1. **Brew a flavorful, sweetened turmeric and cardamom tea**
   Boil 2 quarts of water stirring in the sugar and herbs. Simmer for 10 minutes.

   Add citrus juice.

   Add 2 quarts cold water to cool the mixture.

   Cool the mixture to lukewarm or room temperature.

2. **Add Micro-Organisms (Culture)**
   Add the culture into the cooled tea and stir well.

   (If you are using the ginger bug and want to perpetuate it, see the ginger beer recipe for instructions.)

3. **Bottle and Ferment**
   Strain mixture into a bucket or jar.

   For nonalcoholic soda, you will want to bottle it soon. Funnel mixture into bottles and seal them. Let the bottles sit at room temperature for at least 4 days. Check the bottles daily by burping them, and move to the fridge when they start to get carbonated. This may take up to 10 days or so, depending which culture you used or how active your culture was when you added it.

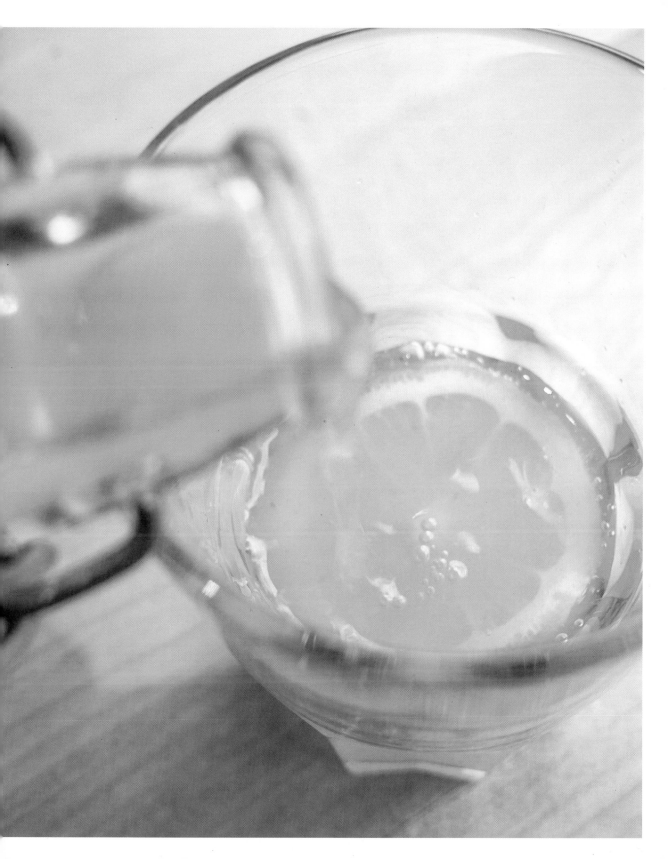

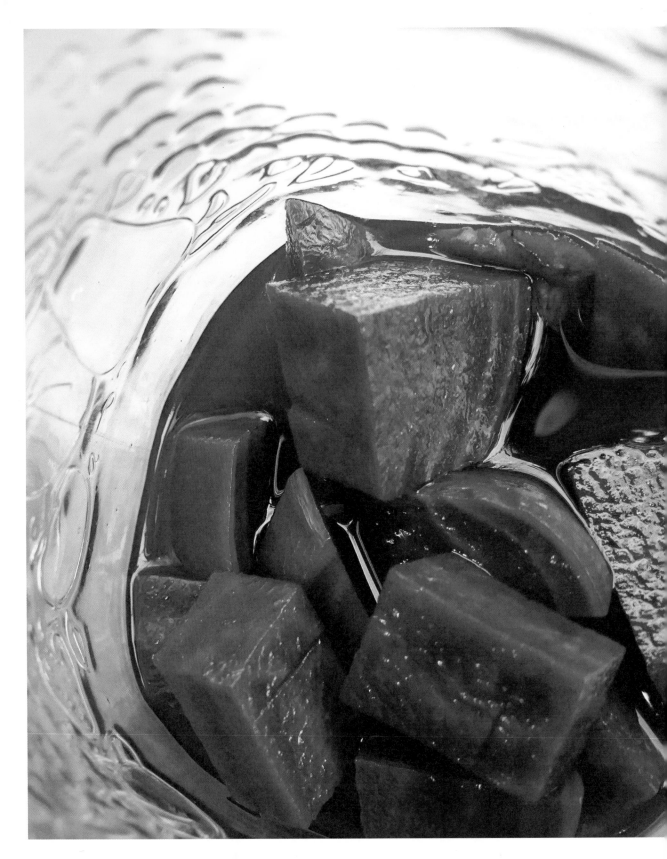

BEET CREAM SODA

Recreate this childhood favorite, but by adding beets instead of col-
oring, and fermenting it instead of just carbonating corn syrup, you'll
make a more sophisticated beverage. Beets contain anthocyanins,
which give them their red color. These antioxidants benefit cardiovas-
cular health.

EQUIPMENT

A pot with at least 4 quarts
    (4 L) capacity
Funnel
Strainer
Measuring cups
Wooden spoon or spatula
Swing-top glass beer bottles to
    4 quarts total capacity
4-quart jar or bucket
Cloth with rubber band to cover

jar or bucket (optional: if you
    want to produce more alcohol)

INGREDIENTS

Water (2 quarts + 2 quarts)
1½ cups sugar
1 medium beet, diced into
    1-inch cubes
1 vanilla pod, split in half
Juice of 1 lemon

Culture options (choose one):
Active ginger bug: use about
    ¼ cup strained volume
Or use 1 cup whey from coconut
    kefir or dairy kefir
Or use 3–5 tablespoons water kefir
    grains (spare or backup ones—
    water kefir grains prefer plain
    water and sugar, but can be
    cycled through to make a batch
    of root beer from time to time)

Directions

1. **Brew a flavorful, sweetened beet and vanilla tea:**
   Wash, peel and dice beet. Split vanilla pod in half, scraping out the
   tiny seeds with the edge of a knife. In the pot, add 2 quarts water,
   sugar, vanilla, and beets. Simmer for 10 minutes.
       Add citrus juice.
       Add 2 quarts cold water to cool the mixture.
       Cool the mixture to lukewarm or room temperature.

◄ Beets in sugar solution for beet cream soda. HONAMI WATANABI

2. **Add Micro-Organisms (Culture)**

Add the culture into the cooled tea and stir well.

(If you are using the ginger bug and want to perpetuate it, see the ginger beer recipe for instructions.)

3. **Bottle and Ferment**

Strain mixture into a bucket or jar.

Be thrifty: you can save the vanilla pod and add it to a jar of sugar. A couple of weeks later, you have vanilla sugar for use in other sodas or baking. While you are at it, you can save those strained beets to snack on or add to a salad.

For nonalcoholic soda, you will want to bottle it soon. Funnel mixture into bottles and seal them. Let the bottles sit at room temperature for at least 4 days. Check the bottles daily by burping them, and move to the fridge when they start to get carbonated. This may take up to 10 days or so, depending which culture you used or how active your culture was when you added it. Be patient.

GINGER BEER AND GINGER BUG FERMENTED SODA TROUBLESHOOTING AND FAQ

1. **Soda does not carbonate**

   Check the seals on the bottles.

   Was the ginger bug active? It should be bubbly and smell yeasty on the day it was added to your brewed soda mixture. If it was only a little active, it will eventually carbonate, just gently shake the bottles and be patient—they will fizz.

   Was the ginger bug added to hot liquid? Oops—that kills the yeast! You'll need to start over.

   Was it fermented in a cold area? Fermentation takes longer or may not even start if it's too cold. Comfortable room temperature and a reasonably steady temperature are key.

   See the section on carbonation in the Chapter 1 for more details.

2. **Bottles explode or geyser when you open them**

   Duck and run for cover! Okay, proceed with caution, but try to move the bottles to a cooler spot. Refrigerate them for a few hours and the carbonation will be more manageable.

   In the future, ferment bottles in a cooler spot or for less time, burp them regularly, and move them to the fridge once they start to carbonate.

   See the section on carbonation in the Chapter 1 for more details.

3. **White film floating on ginger beer**

   That thin white film is a yeast called kham. It's normal and totally fine to drink and happens in some batches naturally. If you are put off by it, discard that batch.

   Sometimes the carbonation/bubbles will gather in patches and look white. Just examine them and make sure it's not mold.

   If it is fuzzy or evidently moldy, throw it out!

4. **How long is it good for? How do I know if it is bad or off?**

    Because fermented beverages are essentially preserved, they can last for months in cool storage. Note, however, that they continue to carbonate in the bottle, so to minimize risk of an explosion, let the pressure off regularly, keep the bottle refrigerated after it carbonates, and try to drink it within a couple of weeks.

5. **How to control and measure alcohol levels**

    Bottling the soda mixture soon after you add the culture will minimize alcohol levels.

    Filling the bottle to halfway up the neck of the bottle (rather than leaving it partly empty) will also minimize alcohol levels.

    Levels of alcohol produced depend on the wild yeast you catch in the ginger bug. If you want to measure alcohol content, you can use a hydrometer, available at beer homebrew supply shops.

6

WHEY-FERMENTED DRINKS

WHEY IS CONSIDERED a byproduct of making cheese; using it to make healthier, probiotic sodas is easy.

There really is a lot of transferability here—you can use whey instead of any other culture to create fizz as well as some additional beneficial bacteria and enzymes that boost digestion. You can choose the ginger beer recipe, for example, and use whey to ferment the soda instead of active ginger bug. Whey can ferment lemonade to make it naturally fizzy, plus you can add it to nearly any other fruit juice to carbonate it.

USING WHEY AS A STARTER FOR FERMENTED SODAS

To substitute whey for another culture, generally, use ¼ cup of whey for every 1 quart of soda you are making.

HOW TO OBTAIN WHEY

The whey from dairy kefir makes the fizziest sodas, due to the naturally high amount of yeast cultures in it. If you make dairy kefir at home, you will have probably taken a batch too far, noticing that the curds separated from the whey. When this happens, just strain the curds out through a few layers of cheesecloth and hang it to drip. The liquid that drips from this coagulated milk is the whey. It is a clear, yellowish color.

Non-dairy cultured coconut kefir (see coconut kefir recipe on page 83) and other non-dairy kefir yogurts may also create delicious curds (strain to make non-dairy cream cheeses!), and you can collect the whey from them.

The whey strained from store-bought, unsweetened yogurt may also be used. Yogurt makes mildly fizzy sodas, but lacks the yeast population that kefir contains, resulting in less carbonation.

The cheesemaking process results in a lot of whey.

Pure whey, free from milk solids, keeps for months in the fridge or can be frozen.

BEET KVASS
RECIPE

EQUIPMENT

1-quart (1L) jar

Lid for jar or tightly woven
  cloth and a rubber band
  to secure it

Measuring cups and spoons

INGREDIENTS

1 medium beet, cleaned and
  chopped into bite-sized
  pieces

Filtered water, a little less
  than 1 quart

½ tablespoon unrefined salt

2 tablespoons–¼ cup whey

As a savory fermented drink, this recipe is a departure from other drinks in this book. It is basically pickled beet tonic, and is really refreshing. Kvass drinks can be made from various vegetables and fruits; there is even a variation that uses stale sourdough bread and sourdough starter. Their salty, sour kvass tonics are much beloved by Russians. After having made this in a fermented beverages workshop, one of the participants had a strong memory of her grandmother making a similar drink. She is Korean, and her grandma would make this slightly salty, somewhat fizzy vegetable juice in the winter. Instead of beets, she used Korean radish, similar to daikon aka LoBok or white radish.

TIP I recommend eating the beets once the kvass has fermented. A tasty byproduct of making kvass is that you get whey-pickled veggies to add to salads, snack on, or add to soups.

Directions

1. Wash beet, cut into bite-sized pieces, and add to the jar.
2. Add other ingredients and shake to combine.
3. Let ferment at room temperature either with a lid loosely on the jar, or with a cloth cover secured with a rubber band.
4. Ferment for at least 2 days, or 4 if you like it more sour.
5. You can decant the kvass and bottle, storing the bottles at room temperature for a couple more days if you like it somewhat fizzy. Refrigerate once decanted and/or carbonated.

Variations

- Add some slices of ginger, a clove of garlic (or both!).
- Add a slice of orange.
- Try this with carrots, daikon, or other root vegetables.

▶ Large-diced beets provide the natural sugars for fermentation of this sour probiotic drink. HONAMI WATANABE

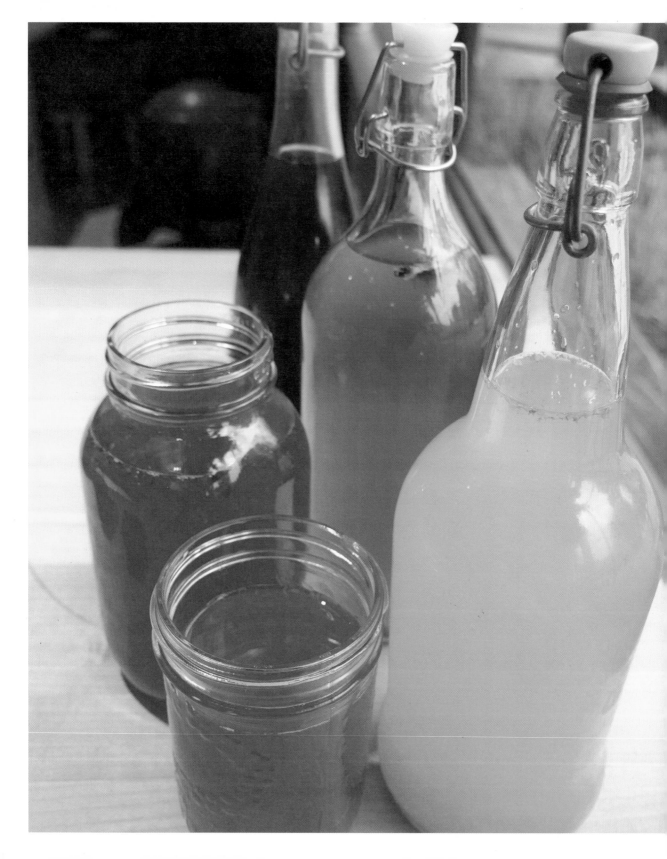

RESOURCES

Cultures for fermentation can be ordered online from

- GEM Cultures: www.gemcultures.com
- Cultures for Health: www.culturesforhealth.com
- Unity Jun (fresh Jun SCOBY including everything you need to brew): www.unityjun.com
- Happy Herbalist: www.happyherbalist.com

Quality herbs, teas, and more can be ordered online from

- Mountain Rose Herbs: www.mountainroseherbs.com
- Harmonic Arts: www.harmonicarts.ca

ABOUT THE AUTHOR

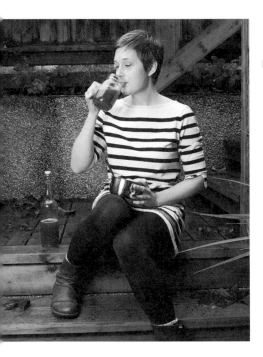

ANDREA POTTER IS a chef and Registered Holistic Nutritionist. She has a background in culinary arts, with Red Seal certification. Since 2009, she has owned and operated Rooted Nutrition, aimed at providing nutrition education to a wide variety of clients. She has taught extensively on topics from whole foods nutrition and alternative baking (including sugar-free, gluten-free, and vegan), to seasonal soups, and fermenting and preserving food. Andrea is passionate about supporting health-motivated cooks to make informed healthy choices that start with vibrant, delicious, practical recipes and culinary techniques.

Learn more at www.rootednutrition.ca

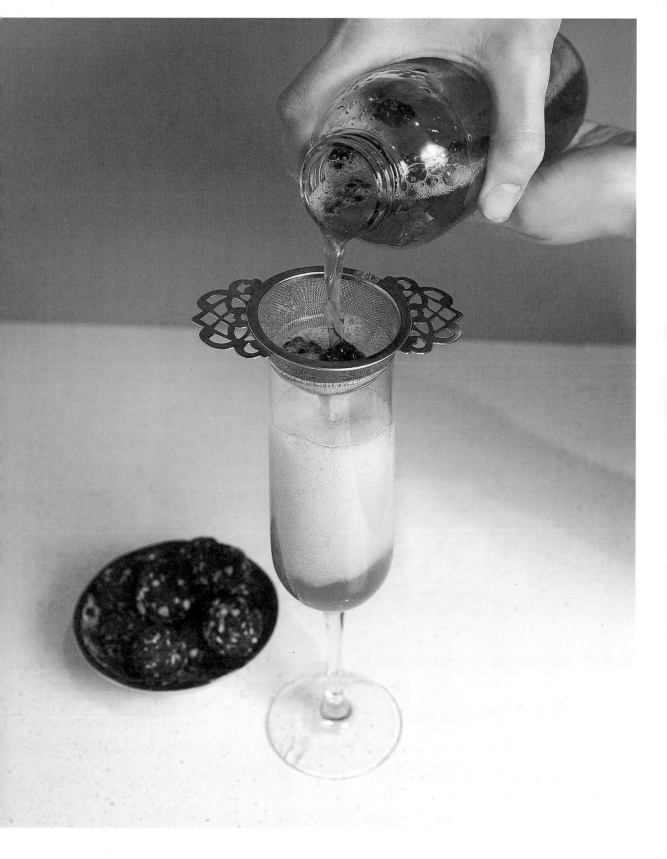

A NOTE ABOUT THE PUBLISHER

New Society Publishers is an activist, solutions-oriented publisher focused on publishing books for a world of change. Our books offer tips, tools, and insights from leading experts in sustainable building, homesteading, climate change, environment, conscientious commerce, renewable energy, and more—positive solutions for troubled times.

We're proud to hold to the highest environmental and social standards of any publisher in North America. This is why some of our books might cost a little more. We think it's worth it!

- We print all our books in North America, never overseas
- All our books are printed on **100% post-consumer recycled paper,** processed chlorine free, with low-VOC vegetable-based inks (since 2002)
- Our corporate structure is an innovative employee shareholder agreement, so we're one-third employee-owned (since 2015)
- We're carbon-neutral (since 2006)
- We're certified as a B Corporation (since 2016)

At New Society Publishers, we care deeply about *what* we publish— but also about *how* we do business.

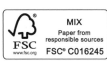

MIX
Paper from
responsible sources
FSC® C016245

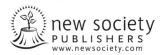
new society
PUBLISHERS
www.newsociety.com

New Society Publishers
ENVIRONMENTAL BENEFITS STATEMENT

For every 5,000 books printed, New Society saves the following resources:[1]

30	Trees
2,695	Pounds of Solid Waste
2,965	Gallons of Water
3,867	Kilowatt Hours of Electricity
4,899	Pounds of Greenhouse Gases
12	Pounds of HAPs, VOCs, and AOX Combined
7	Cubic Yards of Landfill Space

[1]Environmental benefits are calculated based on research done by the Environmental Defense Fund and other members of the Paper Task Force who study the environmental impacts of the paper industry.